Mysticism in the Village

BILL ALLARD

• Canada • UK • Ireland • USA •

Note for Librarians: A cataloguing record for this book is available from Library and Archives Canada at www.collectionscanada.ca/amicus/index-e.html
ISBN 1-4120-8517-9

Printed on paper with minimum 30% recycled fibre. Trafford's print shop
runs on "green energy" from solar, wind and other environmentally-friendly power sources.

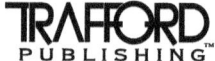

PUBLISHING™
Offices in Canada, USA, Ireland and UK
This book was published *on-demand* in cooperation with Trafford Publishing. On-demand publishing is a unique process and service of making a book available for retail sale to the public taking advantage of on-demand manufacturing and Internet marketing. On-demand publishing includes promotions, retail sales, manufacturing, order fulfilment, accounting and collecting royalties on behalf of the author.

Book sales for North America and international:
Trafford Publishing, 6E–2333 Government St.,
Victoria, BC v8t 4p4 CANADA
phone 250 383 6864 (toll-free 1 888 232 4444)
fax 250 383 6804; email to orders@trafford.com
Book sales in Europe:
Trafford Publishing (uk) Limited, 9 Park End Street, 2nd Floor
Oxford, UK ox1 1hh UNITED KINGDOM
phone 44 (0)1865 722 113 (local rate 0845 230 9601)
facsimile 44 (0)1865 722 868; info.uk@trafford.com
Order online at:
trafford.com/06-0272

10 9 8 7 6 5 4 3 2

Mysticism in the Village

I dedicate this book to Christine.

I acknowledge Fata Mullinax for her editorial assistance.

I will donate 50% of all author book sales royalties to the Unity Church towards the construction of the new Spiritual Life Center and for their silent Unity Prayer Ministry located in Unity Village, Missouri.

-Bill Allard

Chapter 1

SHE MIGHT DIE.

I sat nervously in the waiting room at Bayfront Hospital, hoping for good news about my fiancée, Christine Kolb. We'd become engaged just five days ago on New Year's Eve, and should have been making wedding plans. Instead, we were waiting for the biopsy results from a lump in Christine's breast.

I stared sightlessly at the book I'd been trying to read while trying in vain to ignore my churning stomach. A nurse approached the ever-changing group of worried relatives and friends, then looked around the room with an air of passive sadness. Conversations hushed abruptly as everyone waited for possible news of their loved ones.

"Mr. Allard?" She called my name gently.

"Right here," I answered. I had to stand up slowly; waves

of nausea made me wonder if I could walk. I finally managed to pick up my book and turned to face the nurse.

"Follow me, please." She turned briskly on one crepe-soled heel and led me down a hallway, then through a door to the post-op area. What a dismal place! There were stretchers everywhere, all filled with people crying and moaning.

Gee, this is great, I thought. *I'm in Hell.*

The nurse motioned me into a small cubicle that looked like it was right out of the television series *ER*. Christine was sitting in a chair in the corner, looking drained and tired. That was hardly surprising; after all, the doctor had just taken a chunk of flesh out of her body.

"Hello, sweetheart," I leaned down to kiss her, feeling awkward and afraid my touch might cause her further pain.

Christine smiled weakly and seemed happy to see me, despite her recent ordeal.

I was trying to think of something uplifting to say when Dr. Leslie Pearlstein and his assistant, Melanie Elmore, walked into the cubicle. There was barely enough room for all of us in the sterile, cramped space. I backed out of the way and studied their faces; there were no smiles.

Dr. Pearlstein turned deep, sorrowful eyes to the woman I wanted to marry and said four words I will never forget. "Christine, you have cancer."

Time seemed to stand still in the terrible, hollow silence. My knees became very shaky, and I thought I was actually going to fall over. *My God, what a thing to be told*, I thought with horror.

I composed myself enough to look at Christine. Her face was frozen in shock. Then, I watched the full impact of each word hit her like a bullet; her stoic expression dissolved and she began to cry.

"Am I going to die?" Her voice was a wail of terror.

But Dr. Pearlstein was shaking his head. "You have cancer," he said matter-of-factly. "It does *not* necessarily mean that you're going to die. There are quite a few treatments available, and many are very successful in treating your type of condition."

This encouraging news did not stop her tears. The doctor and his assistant hugged Christine in a vain attempt at comfort, made more reassuring noises, and told her to call the office next week when all the test results would be in.

"In the meantime, try not to worry," Dr. Pearlstein added. "I'll call you as soon as I get the results back from the lab."

After they left, another wave of anxiety washed over me as I turned back to Christine. She had shrunk back into the corner, curled up and shaking like a beaten puppy. She looked up at me with searching eyes and asked desperately, "Bill, what am I going to do?"

I didn't have a clue. I was still in total shock. Cancer: such a bad, scary word. Was she going to die? The whole thing seemed too intense for me to handle. All I could think of was to get her out of this place as quickly as possible.

Forcing a smile, I held out my hand and said softly, "Come on, honey. Let's blow this pop stand. Everything's going to be all right...somehow."

I don't think she believed me, but her fingers closed around mine eagerly and she seemed more than eager to escape from this medical hellhole. I helped her get dressed while the nurse processed her out of the surgery center.

It was a slow, quiet drive home as each of us pondered the same question: *What will happen now?*

The next few days seemed endless as we waited for the results. Christine was still sore from the procedure, so her activities were limited. The enforced rest turned her into a restless cat on a hot tin roof. Imbibing in some good wine seemed like a good solution to take the edge off, and we spent a good deal of time looking at each other wistfully over our goblets. Unfortunately, we had one more health issue to deal with; I was also scheduled for some tests within the next few days to determine if I had colon cancer.

What a first week of the year this had turned out to be!

Chapter 2

IT ALL STARTED JUST A week before, on New Year's Eve. Christine was under the delusion that we didn't have any particular plans, but I had something up my sleeve so special that I was about to explode with anticipation. My friend Dimitri was in town for the holiday and didn't have a date for the evening, so I tried to come up with an idea that wouldn't make him feel like a fifth wheel. We planned to cook dinner at Christine's home first, and then go to a popular local hangout called Philthy Phil's for cocktails and live music.

Dimitri and I arrived at Christine's house around six, and the three of us had a festive time drinking wine and preparing a delicious rack of lamb. In fact, we were enjoying ourselves so much that we wondered if we were going to make it out the door. Though I was having fun, my secret was burning a hole inside of me.

Finally, at ten o'clock, I announced, "Guys, if we don't leave now, we won't make it by midnight."

I breathed a sigh of relief as Christine locked the door behind us and we headed down the street. *We'd better get there in time*, I worried, *everything depends on it.*

The restaurant was only a ten-minute walk; before we knew it, we were at a table in front of the band.

I turned to Christine. "Will you dance with me?"

She smiled, and then walked into my arms.

After a few minutes, I asked, "Having a good time?"

"Oh, yes," she purred blissfully, snuggling closer.

I swallowed hard. "Is there a song you'd like to hear?"

She thought for a moment, grinned, and then grabbed my crotch playfully. "How about Jimmy Buffett's 'A Pirate Looks at Forty?'"

I laughed. After our dance was over, I excused myself and made my way to the stage while the band was between sets and motioned to the lead singer: a classic, old stoner who looked like a pirate himself.

He leaned down and cupped a hand to his ear. "What can I do for you, dude?"

"I want to request a song."

"Sure," he said with a grin. "What would you like to hear?"

"Do you know Buffett's 'A Pirate Looks at Forty?'"

He looked at me as if I'd asked if he knew his ABCs "Of course, dude."

"Great. But this is a *special* request," I told him. "I want you to play it right after 'Auld Lang Syne' at midnight."

The pirate scratched his head. "I don't know. I mean, we'll be happy to play the song, but I really can't guarantee when."

I pulled a twenty-dollar bill out of my pocket and held it

out discreetly. "Look, do you see that blonde over there?" I motioned toward our table, where Christine was talking with Dimitri.

"Sure do. She's fine," he said admiringly.

"Yes, she is—and it's really, *really* important that you play the song then. I'm going to ask her to marry me."

He reached out and deftly took the twenty. "No problem, my friend," he assured me with a wink. "Consider it done."

I made my way back to the table, feeling very proud of myself.

But Dimitri had some bad news. "Look, I'm getting bored," he told me. "Why don't I take off and catch up with you and Christine later?"

Over my dead body, I thought. "You can't," I said flatly.

My friend raised a quizzical eyebrow. "Why not?" he demanded. "Everyone here has a date tonight, and there aren't any single chicks for me to talk to."

"Well, you can't leave yet. I'm planning a big surprise. Besides, I brought along a little something special for you."

This piqued his interest. "Special, huh? It had better be what I hope it is, or I'm getting a cab."

I laughed. "Don't worry—you won't be disappointed. Let's go outside."

After a quick check to make sure Christine was okay, we walked across the street to a restaurant that was closed for the evening and stopped in the shadow of their parking garage. When we were out of view, I pulled out a big fatty.

"Happy New Year," said Dimitri.

"Indeed," I agreed.

By the time we finished our holiday smoke, we were both laughing.

"So, what's this surprise you mentioned?" he asked.

I reached into my pocket, brought out a small, black velvet box, and handed it to him.

"Why, Bill," Dimitri teased, "this is so sudden."

"It's for Christine, dude. Open it!"

When he did, the sparkle of the brilliant round cut, two-carat diamond ring almost blinded him. "Holy shit!" he exclaimed. "This looks serious."

"It is," I said. "That's why I couldn't let you leave. The big moment goes down right after midnight." I dug my camera out of my back pocket and held it out to him. "Do you think you could take a picture of us?"

"Of course." He grinned as he handed back the ring and took the camera. "By the way, congratulations."

"She hasn't said 'yes' yet." I looked at my watch; it was a quarter to twelve. "Time to go back, pal."

We walked back to Philthy Phil's. The band was playing, and Christine was talking to the people at the next table. I sat down with her and kept a nervous eye on my watch. The waitress came by to give everyone a glass of champagne for the midnight toast as the television came on, showing all the people partying in New York. Within moments, the ball dropped in Times Square and everyone screamed, "Happy New Year!"

I turned to Christine and we embraced, followed by a long, deep kiss as the band began to play *Auld Lang Syne*.

"Come with me," I whispered, walking her to the dance floor.

When the song was over, the band's lead singer announced, "And now, here's a special request for a special lady." They began to play *A Pirate Looks at Forty*.

She smiled and kissed me again.

As we began to dance, the singer announced, "Will everyone please clear the floor?"

That twenty bucks had evidently bought me the V.I.P treatment. I stopped dancing, got down on one knee, pulled the box from my pocket, and took out the ring.

Christine's jaw almost hit the floor.

I took a deep breath. Looking into her eyes, I asked, "Will you marry me?"

She just stood there, her mouth still open.

"Well, yes or no?" I asked again.

She finally managed to speak. "Yes!"

Amid loud applause from the crowd, Dimitri took the photograph of our Kodak moment before he disappeared discreetly into the night. Christine and I ascended into a state of total bliss.

The next day was January 1, the first day of the New Year. We spent the time making phone calls and spreading the good word about our engagement. Christine had surgery scheduled for that Friday, January 5th, but it was merely to remove what looked like a benign cyst. Little did we know that what we thought was going to be an easy ride was about to become a plunge into a giant challenge.

Chapter 3

IT WAS SUNDAY, JANUARY 7TH, and the fact that Christine had cancer was beginning to sink in. I began to feel cold and scared inside. Adding to the anxiety was anticipation of my colonoscopy, scheduled for the next day. For those who haven't seen this procedure demonstrated on television on *Today's* terminally perky Katie Couric, it involves sticking a tube with a tiny camera up your ass to see if you have cancerous polyps in your colon. If you do, the nasty critters are snipped off by another handy device at the end of the probe. This test was deemed necessary by my doctor because blood was found in my stool sample during an annual checkup a couple of weeks back.

I tried desperately to deter him from entering my *sanctum sanctorum*. "Look, the blood's probably there because I'm so nervous about proposing to Christine. It's just a hemorrhoid."

From my doctor's expression, I knew it was pointless to argue. He folded his arms and said firmly, "That might very well be true, Bill. However, we'll have it done anyway, just to make sure."

What's this "we" stuff? I thought resentfully. *I'm the one getting reamed, not you.*

I was forbidden to eat anything the whole day before the procedure. Instead, I was to chug a disgusting-tasting liquid that would make me shit all day. I have to take my hat off—or my pants, in this case—to the sadistic people who formulated this stuff. I spent the whole day running between the couch and the toilet, reflecting on the effort required to hold my butt cheeks together long enough to make it to the can before crapping my pants.

While I was spending all this quality time on the porcelain throne, one sobering thought kept recurring: *What if I have cancer, too?* Christine and I were similar in many ways when it came to taste, personal habits, and pet peeves, but this was one time I didn't want to be like her. The day crept by in physical and mental agony dealing with the fact that my fiancée had cancer, and desperately hoping I didn't.

Bright and early on Monday morning, I found myself in the very same pre-op room Christine had been wheeled into the week before. The nurse recognized us from our previous visit, and was very friendly.

Of course she's friendly, I thought bitterly, *we're becoming two of her best customers.* I took off my clothes; put on one of those awful gowns that destroys the last remains of human dignity, and got up on the gurney.

"Everything's going to be all right," Christine said, looking down at me tenderly.

It felt strange to be the one getting all the attention. My new fiancée was facing cancer, yet here she was, taking care of me. The love shining in her eyes made me realize again why I loved this woman so deeply.

The nurse approached with a smile and a metal tray. "Sorry to break this up, but it's time to give you some happy drugs."

Christine kissed me. "I'll see you in a couple of hours."

Soon, another nurse showed up who looked like a professional wrestler and announced gruffly, "We're ready for you now." This brawny angel of mercy grabbed my cart and rolled it briskly down the hallway to the operating room. By this time, everything was beginning to look very fuzzy. In the OR, two more nurses were waiting. Everything they said seemed incredibly funny, and I was still laughing when the doctor showed up. That's the last thing I remember.

When I awoke, my first thought was, *what did they find?*

I didn't have long to wait. The doctor arrived and got right to the point: "I didn't see anything that looked like cancer. As a matter of fact, you seem to be in real good shape up there."

I never thought I'd be willing to kiss a man for telling me I have a nice-looking asshole, but would have been willing to make an exception in this case. "Thank you, thank you, thank you," I blabbered.

Shortly afterward, Christine showed up and shared in my elation at the good news. I was still as high as a kite when she took me out of there, in more ways than one. The ride back home was pleasant, and Christine lovingly tucked me into bed.

Another high-stress day had come to an end.

Tuesday was a mixture of conflicting emotions: relief that my test was negative, anxiety about waiting for Christine's lab results. We jumped each time the telephone rang. The call finally came, and it wasn't good. She definitely had an active cancer, and we were to come in and discuss it with Dr. Pearlstein. An appointment was made for the next day.

Only ten days had elapsed since I got down on one knee on the dance floor at Philthy Phil's and asked Christine to be my wife. Since then, our lives had been a roller coaster of emotions from the incredible high of New Year's Eve and New Year's Day, to the abysmal low of finding out about her cancer. There was an eerie feeling of looking into the great unknown as we headed for the doctor's office to find out exactly what we were facing. I put my arm around Christine as we walked slowly to the elevator. When we reached Dr. Pearlstein's office, I looked at the other waiting patients and thought, *so this is the cancer room. Will it be a place of impending death, or of healing?*

At the moment, it seemed like a room of terror. Christine signed in, sat down, and picked up a magazine. I couldn't read anything. In an attempt to get a grip on my emotions, I closed my eyes and tried to meditate on something more pleasant and discovered that it's very hard to find your "happy place" when you're scared shitless. Fortunately, it wasn't long before Christine's name was called and we were escorted to Dr. Pearlstein's office, where he and his assistant were already waiting.

When we were seated, Dr. Pearlstein said, "Christine, you strike me as a person who likes to know the straight scoop. Am I right?"

She nodded. "Just tell me what's wrong, please."

"All right. To sum it up, you have a stage three, inflammatory, aggressive cancer."

I don't know what that is, but it doesn't sound good, I thought.

There was a pause before Christine asked calmly, "Tell me about it. What does that mean?"

Dr. Pearlstein explained there are basically four stages of

cancer. Stage one is the least invasive; four is the worst. Stage three, then, was obviously pretty bad. The tumor he'd removed had been about the size of a tennis ball. Unfortunately, there had been strands of cancerous tissue on the ends of the mass, which meant the disease was still active.

"You don't have to die from this," he was quick to assure her, "but we do need to discuss treatment as soon as possible. I can arrange for a second opinion, of course, but we recommend that you start chemotherapy immediately."

The doctor and his assistant went on to explain varying recommended options. There would be numerous surgeries, radiation therapy in addition to the chemo, and too many other unpleasant things to recall.

"I can refer you to Dr. Richard Knipe for your chemotherapy," Dr. Pearlstein added. "He's an excellent oncologist. Busy man, though. Let me see if I can set up an appointment for you." He reached for the phone and made a quick call, scribbled some notes, then turned back to Christine. "They can see you right now, if you hurry. Here's the address."

We left the surgeon's office feeling a conflicting mixture of despair amid glimmers of hope. The oncologist's office was only about ten minutes away; before we knew it, we were walking into yet another cancer waiting room. This one was filled with a sea of long, sad faces of patients with bald heads; the ladies were obviously wearing wigs.

I looked at Christine; I could imagine what she was thinking. *'How long will it be before I look like this, too?'*

It seemed like an eternity before her name was finally called and we went in together. I sat quietly by while Dr. Knipe asked numerous questions. After a brief exam, he excused himself to review the lab results. During another eternity of waiting, I noted his diploma on the wall: Notre Dame. I was duly impressed, and encouraged by the fact that this guy probably knew what he was doing.

The doctor finally returned to announce, "Ms. Kolb, I agree with Dr. Pearlstein. We need to start treatment immediately,"

Christine swallowed hard.

I asked, "What do you mean by 'immediately?'"

His direct gaze met mine. "There is definitely cancer present right now," he said bluntly. "The sooner we begin treatment, the more of a chance we have to save her."

Christine and I looked at each other.

"Let's do it," she said.

Dr. Knipe smiled his approval, checked his schedule, and booked her to begin treatment on Monday. He also did his best to give us hope as he laid out the treatment scenario. Christine seemed relieved to know there was finally something proactive she could do to fight the disease.

I asked Dr. Knipe what I could do to help.

"Quite a bit, actually," he answered promptly. He made several suggestions, including which vitamin and herb supplements would be effective, and what substances to avoid. "A healthy diet and plenty of rest," he concluded, "and no smoking!"

This last warning wasn't really necessary; Christine had stubbed out her last cigarette the day she found out she was ill.

As he talked, both of us began to relax a bit. We sensed that Dr. Knipe was definitely a good man, a healer, and that he wanted to heal Christine. It was about five or six o'clock in the afternoon by the time we walked out of his office. We emerged with a lot more hope than when we'd walked in, and I had renewed respect for oncologists.

We had tickets to *The Phantom of the Opera* for that evening at the Tampa Bay Performing Arts Center. I had purchased them weeks ago, long before what I was beginning to think of as "The Dark Times."

I looked at Christine a bit apprehensively and asked, "Are you still up for tonight?"

She smiled and said without hesitation. "I'm going to make it." Her voice was firm. "We're going to the opera."

On the way, she called her mother on the cell phone to catch her up on the day's events. *Phantom* was a very good performance, and seemed to be the perfect way to take our minds off all the tremendous worry and concern about what was going to happen next.

I remember holding Christine's hand and gazing at her, thinking, *Will she be here a year from today, or will she be dead? It was only ten days ago that I asked her to marry me, and now I'm looking at a person who may die soon.*

I know that sometimes, the best thing is just to live in the moment. Despite the dim prospects, I was happy to be at the opera where I didn't have to talk about it: happy to enjoy the music and performance. This was an evening to hold Christine's hand, put my arm around her, and simply love her.

Unfortunately, I couldn't ignore the immense challenge ahead—and that at that point, I wasn't sure it was a challenge she could meet. My helpless frustration and panic persisted despite the marvelous music and brilliant figures on the stage. *This is bigger than I am.* I despaired, clenching my fists in the dark. *I've always been the kind of guy who can handle any problem, resolve any situation. Roll my sleeves up, jump in, get it done—that's me. But how the hell do I help the woman I love beat this?*

Chapter 4

THE NEXT DAY, WE BOTH went about our business and back to work. I stopped at a Barnes and Noble bookstore on my way home, where I spent about two hours reading bits and pieces from every book on breast cancer I could find. I finally settled on buying seven books that included just about every aspect of the subject: healing yourself with your mind, *The Do's and Don'ts of Breast Cancer*, even one by a doctor who had survived the disease.

The lady at the cash register observed, "Looks like you're going to become an expert on breast cancer."

I met her curious gaze. To my horror, tears welled in my eyes and spilled down my face as I whispered, "I don't know what else to do." My voice was quivering. There I was, crying in the checkout line at Barnes and Noble. Half of me wished the earth would open up and swallow me; the other half was too miserable to care what anyone thought.

The woman stared at me in surprise for a moment. I saw her face soften with pity as she said softly, "I hope it will be okay." She slid the shopping bag toward me across the counter.

"Thanks. Me, too." I grabbed it and hurried out the door.

I reached home and surprised Christine with the books, then got online that night and began researching the Internet for more information. I wanted to see what her odds of survival were, and what we could do to increase them. We began talking candidly about what I learned from the books and the research, though the initial results were not encouraging. For her type of cancer, the odds were sixty percent that she would be dead in a couple of years.

Sixty percent. This was more than one of life's obstacles: it was a mountain. I knew it was time to pray harder than ever before. I couldn't beat this on my own, and didn't think Christine could beat it with just the two of us working on it. We needed help.

Monday arrived, and it was time for the first chemo treatment. Chemotherapy is simply defined thusly: "We will put poison in you to kill the bad things. In the meantime, your body will be very aware that it's being poisoned." Acute nausea, weight loss, hair loss...the list of side effects read like *Vault of Horror* comics. Many of the books I read predicted that chemo would be considered archaic in the years to come, but admitted it was the best thing currently available.

With Christine's fighting spirit, Dr. Knipe's advice and exhaustive research and reading over the past few days, we'd already begun a vitamin program including Tahitian noni juice, and were making radical diet adjustments. We worked together as a team, telling each other that together, we were going to make it. But I was still praying as hard as I could.

We were driving to the first chemo treatment when she told me, "Bill, you didn't have to come."

I laughed. "Yeah? How did you plan to get home afterward?"

"Oh, I'd be able to do it."

"That's not what I've heard about this stuff." I shook my head slowly.

She caught my eye at a red light. "Honey, I can't die. Matthew needs a mother."

Matthew was Christine's four-year-old son. He was in preschool, and a bright, happy little fellow. I sighed. Yes, he certainly did need his mommy.

We arrived at a large building next to St. Anthony's Hospital and walked into an outpatient chemotherapy treatment center, which I quickly came to refer to as "Chemoland." The room was filled with about fifteen or sixteen lounge chairs, scattered in various places. There were televisions for entertainment, and quiet little corners for seclusion. Some of the chairs were occupied by smiling people who looked as if they were getting better. Others wept while curled into the fetal position, immersed in their private agony as they skirted the edge of death.

It was a graphic illustration of what these chemicals can do to the human body, and I wondered how many of these poor souls would be there on our next visit. It also brought me face-to-face with the possibility that the treatment could kill Christine before the cancer did.

I prayed silently, *God, please help me!*

Cancer. We didn't like to call it that. We liked to call it

"Christine's condition," or "Christine's health challenge." But whatever the terminology, it was still cancer.

Though Chemoland was not a happy place, I soon noticed hope in the eyes of many of the patients, largely due to the care of the excellent nurses. They were cheerful, loving, caring, and did their best to bring some light into the shadow of impending death.

Christine was readied for her ride of a lifetime via what they call a "port" put into her chest, an IV, then anti-nausea drugs to keep her from puking her guts out right off the bat. It must not have been successful all the time; there were plenty of bathrooms, and I saw more than a few people hurry into them. We sat there for three or four hours as the chemicals dripped into her veins.

I had to use one of those restrooms after a while myself; it felt as if my insides were coming out from all the stress.

In an attempt to distract myself from the oppressive atmosphere at Chemoland, I read a lot of magazines. Often, I'd finally get absorbed in an article when one of the patients would start wailing, "I can't take it! I can't take it any more! I'd rather die!"

At first, I would lift my head and watch the nurse rush over to comfort the distressed patient. After a while, I just kept reading.

There were exceptions, however. One afternoon I saw a man walk over to one of the nurses and ask, "Is my son okay over there?" He gestured toward a fifteen-year-old boy who was withered away to almost nothing.

The nurse smiled and replied brightly, "Oh, he's fine. He's still receiving his treatment."

The distraught parent asked a little too loudly, "Is he just sleeping…or is he dead?"

The bright voice took a lower tone, "Sir, please. He's just sleeping."

The father looked at her blankly, turned, and walked out of the room weeping.

This was just a taste of what life—or rather, the fight against death—was like in Chemoland. It became difficult just to walk in the door after the first few visits. When it was time to go, I left any reading material I had brought with me under the pretense that maybe someone else might enjoy what I had abandoned. The truth was, anything that had been in that awful room felt somehow contaminated. I just wanted to leave the smell, taste and texture of the whole experience back among the lounge chairs. In fact, nothing in the world would have compelled me to go back there...except Christine.

After her first treatment, she had a hard time getting out of the lounge chair. We walked very slowly out of the building. I got her into the car and drove her home.

Despite her weakness, she was relatively okay the first day. She was even able to eat a little soup before she went to bed. I stayed at her home, watching over her and getting Matthew to bed.

"What's wrong with Mommy?" he asked as I tucked him in.

I tried to make light of the matter. "Well, pal, Mommy wasn't feeling too good today. She's a little sick, but she's going to feel better."

Fortunately, that seemed to satisfy him, at least for the moment.

That was Day One.

On Day Two, Christine's condition rapidly deteriorated.

Days Three and Four were the worst so far. Anything that had an odor, including food and cooking smells, made her vomit. She was sick all the time. It was torture to see her in this debilitated condition and not know what to do. I consulted more books for ideas to help, and went to the health food store for recommended supplements. It took everything I had to control my worry and also be a good caretaker for Matthew, who had no idea his mother might be dying.

By Day Five, however, the veil lifted a bit. This improvement increased through the next three weeks, until Christine was feeling almost like her old self again. She even returned to work. I knew from reading about chemotherapy that this period was just the calm before the storm, when the poison would really start to kick in. But she shook her head when I suggested she take some time off from work.

"I have a son to take care of. I have to work," she said firmly. "Besides, it takes my mind off the cancer."

It was the night before the second chemo treatment. Christine had been feeling better, and her health seemed to be improving. I was just getting Matthew settled after a long day when she called from the living room, "Bill, would you come in here, please?"

"Be right there," I answered, after kissing Matthew goodnight, I went to see what she needed. Christine made room on the couch, sat up to put her arms around me, then pulled back to look into my eyes.

"This was not part of the deal," she said. To my amazement, she began to remove her engagement ring. "You can take this back. I know you didn't know this was part of the package when you asked me to marry you just a little more than a month ago, and you've already done far more than I expected you to do." She smiled sadly. "It's okay to get off, Bill. You can get off this ride right now, because this is a very, very rough road."

But before she could get the ring off, I pushed it back firmly onto her finger. "No," I said emphatically. "I asked you to marry me. I *want* you to marry me. We're going to beat this cancer together, you're going to get all better, and we're going to get married. You keep that ring on your finger, Christine, and just let me help you."

She hugged me, and we both sat there and cried.

After we both calmed down, we had a long talk. For the first time, I opened up to Christine and confessed that this first treatment made me realize I needed help with the situation. I admitted that taking care of her, Matthew, my business, and trying to keep some sort of continuity in my life had become very difficult.

Christine agreed wholeheartedly. She said she would call her staff and ask them to volunteer to deliver meals the first five days following her treatment. This way I wouldn't have to worry about cooking, and there would be plenty left over from dinner for lunch the next day.

We lined up our schedules. She wanted to work the morning of her second treatment to get as much done as possible. I said I would come by to pick her up later that afternoon. She didn't argue this time; she knew now that she'd be knocked out for the next few days. We were to learn quickly that just when she was feeling better from the last treatment, it was time to go back for another. Her appointment was for 2:00 PM; I pulled up to her house at 1:30, and off we went to Chemoland again.

The nice thing about this trip was that we didn't have to go all the way into downtown St. Petersburg. We were heading for another facility in Pasadena that was much closer to home. The atmosphere was different, too. It had windows overlooking the Intracoastal Waterway, and didn't feel quite as depressing as the first chamber of horrors. We were shown into a smaller room with eight to ten lounge chairs placed in the now-familiar random pattern. We also saw the same bald people, and ladies wearing telltale wigs.

They called us in, weighed and evaluated Christine, and we had another talk with Dr. Knipe. He gave us more encouragement and constructive ideas, and then sent us to the room for Christine's treatment.

I was armed with plenty of magazines, and read quietly until the silence was shattered by a woman's scream.

"I can't take it any more! I can't take it! I feel so sick…I can't take it! I need help!"

The nurse rushed over to a patient who was writhing in agony.

The woman shouted, "I'm going to die soon. I know I'm going to die! Why should I go through the torture of more treatments? Why should I have to do this?"

Holding the sick, sobbing woman in her arms, the nurse rocked her like a child.

I closed my eyes and tried to forget where I was. After the now predictable stressful visit to the bathroom, I walked out to see Christine lying passively in her lounge chair. *She's going to feel just like that woman in the next few weeks*, I reflected. *I hope to God that I can be as strong and supportive as that nurse.*

When Christine had been sufficiently pumped full of poison, they unhooked her and we left. She asked me to get the car and pull it up to the front entrance.

"I don't think I can walk that far," she confessed.

We picked up Matthew from preschool on the way home. He climbed into the car and regarded his mother curiously. "Mommy, are you okay?"

Christine summoned enough strength to say, "I'm fine, Matthew. I'm just a little sick today."

Matthew said, "Mommy, let me kiss you and make you feel better."

He reached over the seat, hugged his mother, and kissed her on the cheek. It was a good thing he couldn't see her tearstained face.

We got home and I was getting Christine ready for the long evening ahead when the doorbell rang. It was one of her salespeople, bringing dinner. I let him in. He seemed very happy to be of help, and very sad to see Christine in such a state. When I walked him out to the car, I was so overcome with gratitude and relief that someone had cared enough to help that I hugged him. I turned away and walked quickly back into the house.

The meal was excellent. Matthew ate plenty, and Christine ate a little before she had to go to bed.

The second day, as expected, she got worse. The third day was another nausea nightmare, but she assured me she was going to be all right. I took her at her word and decided to go to my office. I dropped Matthew off at preschool first, came back to Christine's house to make sure she was okay, got her something to eat, and propped her up with some pillows. I knew it was going to be a rough day and tried to adjust my work schedule accordingly, but my field of investment real estate is a high-pressure one, and trying to keep my mind on work while caring for Christine, Matthew, and cancer was extremely difficult. So, on Day Three of the second chemo, I left the office early. I went home and tried to relax, then went over to Christine's. I found her lying on the floor.

Terrified, I took her in my arms. "Are you all right?"

She opened her eyes and looked up at me sadly. "I'm okay, Bill... I just didn't have the strength to get up off the floor."

I got her back on the couch and realized that things weren't getting better; they were getting worse. Christine was starting to get a bit of a sunken look, and I knew she was having difficulty taking care of herself and her son.

I suggested in mid-February that maybe she should consider moving in with me. It would be much easier to take care of her and Matthew in my home, and I wouldn't have to run back and forth between our two houses.

She pondered the idea. "Well, under these conditions, maybe I should just sell my home."

"No," I said. "Your house is a very good investment, especially out here on the beach. When all this is finished, you'll be happy you still have it. Why don't you give some thought to my finding a tenant to rent it? You can get more than your mortgage payment and have some cash flow. And, " I added, "you can live with me for free."

"I'll think about it," she said quietly.

That evening, the doorbell rang; it was another of her sales associates with food. I put it on the table, and Matthew and I sat down to dinner.

'Christine? Are you going to try to eat?" I called.

She came to the table, smelled the food, ran to the bathroom, and vomited over and over again.

Matthew looked worried. "Is Mommy still sick?"

"Yes," I told him. "But she's going to get better, I promise."

I prayed it was a promise that could be kept.

Christine seemed to be less nauseated by days four and five when another complication reared its ugly head. Chemotherapy depletes the immune system, so one is very susceptible to infection and must avoid exposure to colds and flu. Despite all our precautions Christine developed a persistent cough and a fever.

By day five there was no improvement, and I insisted she get to a doctor. Dr. Knipe wasn't available, but she got an appointment to see one of the other oncologists later that week.

By day seven and eight, she had become independent again and announced she was going to drive to the doctor's office on her own. She did it, too.

That night as I was dishing out dinner I asked her, "What happened?"

"The doctor told me I have pneumonia, and I'm supposed to stay in bed for the next few days."

I could tell from the flatness of her tone that there was more. "Okay, tell me. How bad is it?" I demanded.

She swallowed hard and replied, "If I don't get better in the next two days, he's going to put me in the hospital." Further prodding revealed her physician's concern that she could die from the infection.

I tried to remain calm. "Well, we'll just have to make sure you get better, won't we?" I gave her a reassuring smile and said casually, "Excuse me for just one minute…I have to wash my hands."

I went to the bathroom and closed the door, turned on the water at the sink, and sat on the closed toilet seat. I began to cry. *Oh, my God*, I panicked, *if the chemo doesn't get her, the pneumonia will. How can she possibly survive?*

With control restored at length, I got up and washed my face at the still-running sink. I went back to Christine and said brightly, "Well, if I'm going to take better care of you, I can arrange to take some more time off work and help out."

Christine opened her mouth to say something, then closed it and silently nodded. What was she supposed to say? "Gee, Bill, I'm really sorry I went and got cancer?"

Chapter 5

MATTHEW WAS BEGINNING TO GET a bad cold. By the next day, he was running a high fever and I had two patients on my hands. We called the pediatrician and got an immediate appointment. I watched him play halfheartedly with the toys in the waiting room and reflected dismally, *Christine is at home ill with pneumonia and the effects of chemotherapy and cancer…now I have this sick, trusting little boy to care for.* I closed my eyes and silently prayed, *Please, God, give me the strength to walk this road. Help me to get through this.*

My reverie was interrupted by the nurse's voice. "Mr. Allard? The doctor will see you now."

Good news: Matthew didn't have pneumonia: just a bad cold. The doctor wrote out two prescriptions, and we stopped at the drugstore on the way home to have them filled. While I was getting the sick little guy tucked into bed and making sure he and Christine had taken their meds, the emotional exhaustion caught up with me. *Here I am trying to be the caretaker of these people I love,* I reflected bitterly, *and all I can feel is overwhelmed.*

I went back to check on Christine and found her spread-eagled across the bed, so I grabbed a blanket and went to sleep on the couch. I immediately fell into an exhausted slumber.

Everyone seemed to feel a little better the next day. Matthew soon emerged as good as new and went back to school; Christine survived the pneumonia and went back to work. Finally, I did, too.

It was now mid-to-late February and nearing the date for Christine's third chemo, so she was in the phase of feeling pretty good. Then, the side effect she dreaded most kicked in; her hair began to fall out. One weekend when Matthew was spending the weekend with his father, Tom, she and I confronted the issue.

"I hate this!" she admitted, "but I guess its part of the price of getting better."

I smiled at her positive attitude and announced, "Well, sweetheart, it looks like it's time to go wig shopping."

That Saturday morning we went to The Wig Shop, a small establishment in downtown St. Petersburg. They must have had a thousand different wigs in every imaginable color. I couldn't resist trying one on myself, and jumped out to surprise Christine. She jumped.

"What do you think of this one?" I asked, posing dramatically.

We laughed, and it felt good; laughing wasn't something we'd done much of for a while.

After trying on a few styles, Christine chose a wig very close to her original hair color that was short, attractive, and professional looking. She refused to let me pay for it, insisting her insurance would cover the cost.

"Ah," I said, "but I want to buy you the Saturday night wig."

I could tell by her smile that she knew just the one I meant. It was a long, wild blonde model she'd tried on earlier, and boy, did it look great to me!

She did let me pay for that one, and wore it that night when we went out and had a great time dining and dancing the night away. As I held her in my arms I sensed that somehow, some way, we were going to get through this.

On another evening not long after the wig-buying excursion, I went to Christine's house to help her make dinner, since it was one of the nights we were not scheduled for a delivery from her office staff. She went into the bathroom and came out crying, holding thick strands of hair in her hands.

"I'm losing it all!" she cried.

Shortly after that, she became completely bald. She looked like the poster child for cancer. Her skin began to turn yellow, her face was sunken, and to see her without a wig was scary. We were just a couple of months into this, and already she looked like an inmate in a concentration camp. I could sense her struggle to stay alive and still be a person despite her obvious suffering: her determination to go to work and care for her child, and for me.

I decided a little well-earned diversion might help her odds of winning that struggle. It was getting close to the time for her third chemotherapy session when I told Christine, "We've got a couple of days right now when we know you'll be feeling your best. Why don't we take a quick weekend out to Colorado before your treatment? I know a great place in Glenwood

Springs, and we can put you in the healing waters there. It'll make you all better."

Her face lit up. "That sounds good!"

I got the tickets, and off we flew to Glenwood Springs and a historic spa that had been frequented by Teddy Roosevelt. We enjoyed the therapeutic waters and vapor caves next door, where we inhaled the reputedly healing steam.

Christine was feeling pretty good and announced one morning, "Listen, Bill, I love you, but I can do this without you. Why don't you go up to Aspen today and visit Dimitri?"

I hadn't seen my friend since the night Christine and I had become engaged. After more reassurance from Christine that she would be fine, I gave him a call, then and drove up to Aspen.

It was great to see Dimitri. He got lift tickets and equipment, and we had a great day on the slopes. We came back late in the afternoon and retrieved another friend, then picked up Christine for dinner. Dimitri tried to hide his reaction, but it was obvious he was shocked at the change in her appearance.

Christine held herself together well and seemed to have fun at dinner, but I could see she was tiring quickly. This wasn't unusual; most nights, she couldn't last much past eight o'clock.

Dimitri and his friend were ordering dessert when I faked a yawn and said casually, "Look, guys. Let me pick up the check, but I think we'll head home now. It's been a long day."

Despite the specter of illness, it was a great trip to Colorado. We enjoyed the surroundings, and the act of just getting away somehow made Christine feel more alive and confirmed the fact that she was still somebody. It made her feel real.

When she was in the bathroom the night before we left, Dimitri leaned over to me and whispered anxiously, "Bill, is she getting any better? She looks like she's dying."

I said slowly, "That's because it's possible that she is."

We returned from the Old West to the New South, and St. Petersburg. On March 1, the day after our arrival at home, Christine was scheduled for chemo treatment number three. Ironically, it was also the two-month anniversary of our engagement. What a way to celebrate the occasion: a trip to Chemoland.

I was beginning to be a regular figure at these treatments, and by the third visit had developed a pretty good sense of the way things worked. The first two experiences had been such an emotional shock that I hadn't absorbed much, but this time was different. I recalled that a lot of people brought along snacks and treats, so I stopped at a health food store and bought cashews, muffins, and some salsa and chips. The snacks were a big hit with everyone, including the nurses. I continued to buy magazines, read them, and then left them for everyone to share. Just call me Chemo Claus.

Christine was given her anti-nausea injection, then the chemical drip. We sat there and made the best of it, but she emerged as weak as a newborn kitten.

I got her home, fed, and settled, picked up Matthew and did the same for him before rushing off to Tampa International Airport to pick up my mother, who was flying in from Chicago. Since I was rarely home any more, it was a perfect arrangement for both of us that Mom stay in my usually empty house. We had a nice talk on the drive back from Tampa, and I dropped her off to unpack and settle in before heading back to Christine's for the long night ahead.

Unfortunately, day three was the usual for Christine; she was very ill. We had learned to get anti-nausea injections by day four to control the vomiting, but we had to go to the facility near St. Anthony's Hospital, not the one close to her house. On Sunday morning, March 4, we headed for downtown St. Petersburg's Chemoland. We took the newspaper along and had a jovial time kidding around and laughing during the drive. By now we were over the shock of discovery about Christine's cancer, and were even beginning to make fun of it. We had to; if we didn't laugh about it sometimes, we'd spend all our time crying.

Christine suddenly announced, "I don't know if I'll make it down there, I feel so sick. You might have to pull over before we get there so I can throw up."

"No problem," I said calmly. "I know the program. I'll just pull over to the side of the road, and then you open the door and ralph your guts out. When you're finished, we'll continue on to where we're going."

We eventually made it to Chemoland. Christine got hooked up and had barely started receiving treatment when she had to rush to the bathroom, where she vomited again for about fifteen minutes.

She finally came back out and looked at me balefully. "Well, I guess I didn't get the medication soon enough," she said with a weak laugh.

The anti-nausea medicine started kicking in shortly afterward, and she started to feel better. We eventually were on our way to enjoy the rest of a beautiful Sunday afternoon.

A couple of days later, Christine pulled herself together and we went to a wonderful dinner with our mothers. It turned out to be a fantastic dining experience. Everyone was in good spirits, and Christine kept gazing at me with love and appreciation. She seemed to sense that after a couple of months of this, I was feeling a little rocky. She was right.

Our eyes met across the table. I could see the gleam in hers, and she saw the sparkle in mine as we exchanged an electrifying look of love. We were sitting there with our mothers, but our passion was so strong that but we might as well have been alone. Even the specter of cancer was forgotten in our happiness at being together that evening.

But Christine remembered the shakiness she had sensed in me that night. She suggested a few days later that it might be a good idea that I attend a support group for those caring for cancer patients. I agreed; any help was welcome at this point.

Boy, oh boy, was this an experience! The meeting was early on a Saturday morning, and I walked into a room with fifteen to twenty people sitting around, all talking about what they were dealing with. Some were already crying, and the meeting hadn't even started yet. I resisted the urge to flee and took a seat. Christine wasn't with me; in fact, I think there was only one patient present. They referred to us as "caregivers," and we were encouraged to express our problems and concerns. I listened to many talk about loved ones close to death who'd been told by their doctors that all modern medicine could do was to "make them comfortable."

How do you keep someone 'comfortable' who's getting ready to die? I wondered.

There was one tear-jerking tale after another. When my turn came, I spoke at length about the difficulty of helping Christine by constantly running from my home to hers. The group suggested that I might want to talk to her about moving in. They said it might be a lot easier on both of us, if I was up for it.

"I've talked to her before about it, but she never gives me an answer." I paused, and then smiled at the group. "Thanks. I'll talk to her about it again when I get home."

The meeting was a well-needed eye-opener: seeing the tremors in these people, the despondency in some eyes, and hope in others. There were those who'd reached at the end of their rope as caregivers who were openly hoping for death to release their loved ones. It was a room filled with volatile emotions, and certainly not a place I wanted to be. I was still glad I had been there.

I brought up the subject once more to Christine that evening.

"But why don't we just sell my house, Bill?' she suggested again. "It'll make things simpler, and who knows what's going to happen? I could certainly use the money."

I looked earnestly into her eyes as we sat on the couch. "Sweetheart, you're going to make it. You have a good investment here on the beach. Why don't you let me rent it out? You can have some cash flow on the rent versus your mortgage payment, and as I said before, you can move in with me rent-free. This way, you'll be ahead."

She had to agree that this was not only a good financial decision, but would also take some of the weight off my shoulders. It had obviously become a big emotional drain on me doing all the errands, taking Matthew to school and picking him up, taking Christine to chemotherapy, bringing her home, and generally trying to make sure everybody was all right.

I was happy when she agreed to move in. Besides, we loved each other.

Though I needed more assistance in some areas, we were still getting support in others: my son Erik and his wife, Amanda, were a huge help with Matthew. Many people from Christine's office were still bringing us the very welcome post-chemo meals.

It had been two months since Christine's diagnosis, and we decided it was high time to take a closer look at our spiritual as well as physical well-being. We began contacting every prayer group we could find in the area. Everyone we knew asked everyone they knew to pray for Christine. She began receiving truly touching emails from people praying for her all over the country. The quest for spiritual strength eventually led me to a place called Unity Village, and we began having them pray for Christine through a prayer group they call "Silent Unity." We knew beating cancer was far beyond our abilities and that we needed to enlist a higher authority, a higher source, and a power that could heal.

Chapter 6

THE BIG TOPIC OF DISCUSSION continued to be "the move." We decided to continue our conversation over dinner at Philthy Phil's, where we'd become engaged on New Year's Eve. This time, Matthew joined us. He was a very good boy that evening, despite the fact that he could sense something important was being discussed by the grownups. Christine and I held hands across the table, and agreed that our living together was a major commitment on my part as a caretaker for her and a parent for Matthew.

As we talked, a part of my mind recalled recent advice from well-meaning friends. A lot of them asked me, "Are you sure you're ready for this? It's going to be a lot of work...and it's not exactly what you anticipated when you proposed, is it?" Others played devil's advocate and said, "Come on, Bill. She probably knew she had cancer when you asked her to marry you, and accepted in hopes you'd feel obligated to take care of her."

But I knew in my heart that this woman and I loved each other, and that we were going to make this happen. So on Friday, March 16, Christine arrived with the moving van to bring a feminine touch to my old bachelor's pad.

The next day was St. Patrick's Day. We decided we were due for some time off after all the work of moving, so we took off for a local pub called the Harp and Thistle. We ate corned beef sandwiches and listened to music, danced, hugged, and had a marvelous time. We returned home knowing all was well.

March 18, 2001: the move-in was complete. There really wasn't much adjusting to do; we pretty much fit like a hand in a glove. Christine went about her business; I went about mine, and continued helping with Matthew.

Only a few days later, on Thursday, March 22, it was time for chemotherapy again. This fourth treatment took a terrific toll on Christine; we had to make sure she got enough fluids on Friday, Saturday, and Sunday. There were also shots, monitoring red blood cells, white blood cells…a little bit of everything. My head was spinning with the complexity of it all.

Christine was looking very drawn and gaunt, and had the skin tone of a banana. When we went out to dinner with friends, they waited until she went to the restroom and turned to me, appalled. "She looks so *bad!*" they whispered.

I always smiled and answered, "Well, she's keeping her spirits up, and we're going forward together."

We spent all weekend obsessed with fluids and other medical necessities. This was the first treatment she'd had since we began living together, and I must say it was a lot easier having everything and everyone settled in one place.

The situation with Matthew was also going well. He knew

Mommy was sick, but we were quick to assure him that she was going to get better. The good part was that we were doing quite well together operating as a family. The bad part was that I was still feeling a little beat up and shaken by it all, especially when I saw how Christine looked; it was extremely traumatizing.

On March 22, it was time to go to Moffitt Cancer Center at Tampa's University of South Florida for another opinion. We'd been seeing a local oncologist and surgeon in St. Petersburg, but everyone we talked to strongly suggested we should get all the opinions we could.

Moffitt is considered one of the top cancer centers in the country. I'm sure they do wonderful things for many people, but what a massive, impersonal facility it was! It was like a cancer patient factory where you just felt like one more among the dying. It was a despairing place that just didn't do anything positive for me or for Christine. The team of people we talked to were very nice, checked all our records, and pretty much concluded what Christine's physician had found; what she had was a stage three, aggressive inflammatory cancer. They added that according to their statistics, 60 to 65 percent of patients in her condition died within a couple of years. Not the best prognosis.

We had a long discussion with the Moffitt team about lumpectomy versus mastectomy. The lumpectomy preserved most of the breast, while the mastectomy was a more radical removal that would include not only the breast, but also the surrounding lymph nodes. They recommended a mastectomy, since the cancer was at such an advanced stage. While they didn't really tell us anything we hadn't heard before, it was good to get reinforcement that at least we were being fed the right information.

We left Moffitt and went out for lunch at a health food place near the campus to talk about Christine's options. While sharing my impression about the Moffitt team's knowledge, she also found the atmosphere oppressive. She was feeling a little weak from her last chemo treatment, and I put my arm around her to help her out to the car.

She looked up at me with tears in her eyes. "Thank you for taking the day off to be with me…it means a lot, you know."

"I know," I said hoarsely, and tried to hide my own tears as I gave her a big hug, put her in the car, and took my time walking around to the driver's side to get my emotions under control. *One of us has to be strong,* I thought. *Right now, I guess it had to be me.*

Happier times were on the way, however. Christine's sister and family came to visit a few days before opening day for the St. Petersburg Devil Rays, who were starting the season against Toronto on April 3. It was nice to see Christine perk up, and I was really grateful to have additional help with her care. I got tickets to the game for everyone, including my son Erik, his wife Amanda, and their son, Mitchell. We took some photos, and it was shocking to see how Christine looked after they were developed. She was happy, however, and we had a wonderful family day at the ballpark. Our guests stayed for about a week, and we all had a great time.

Sick though she was, Christine didn't plan to let illness stop her volunteer work with the community. On April 7, we showed up to sell beer at the Festival of States, St. Petersburg's annual week-long celebration. We had the shift from 2:00 till 6:00 P.M. Things started out pretty much by the book, but as we began talking to the other vendors around us and the music began to play, we loosened up considerably. We were soon selling *and* drinking our fine product while having a grand time with everyone. We left promptly at 6:00 for Tampa International Airport to pick up my brother, Ed. My sister, Mary, was also due to arrive the next morning.

The next afternoon Christine announced she was feeling pretty good, so we dropped our pontoon boat in the water for a little marine recreation. The canal behind my house leads to Tampa Bay, and we cruised luxuriously back to the Festival of States in St. Petersburg. It was a fabulous afternoon with my brother, sister, and future wife, whom everyone had already accepted as part of the family.

I was learning from Christine that though one might be ill and facing challenges, life is too expansive to allow such troubles to engulf one's identity. She was still a great person, was doing a good job at work, her company insurance provider was excellent, and her co-workers were going out of their way to be supportive. It really showed me that there is divinity inside each one of us. Sometimes it may take hard times for it to manifest itself, but it is there.

Chapter 7

JUST A SHORT TIME AFTER Ed and Mary left—April 12, to be exact—we had a meeting with Dr. Knipe, Christine's oncologist, and Dr. Pearlstein, her surgeon, It was time to discuss the next step. Both doctors agreed that a radical mastectomy should be performed on the right side where the large tumor was located. Hopefully, that would get all the cancer. Although it was a scary situation, we were relieved at the possibility that surgery would be the end of Christine's ordeal.

Her sister, Jenny, arrived on the day before we took her to the hospital on April 26. The waiting was torture. Jenny and I played pool to pass the time, and then returned to the hospital. The surgery had begun at 10:00 AM; it was nearly 6:00 PM when Dr. Pearlstein finally emerged from the OR.

"Everything went well," he told us. "From what I can see, there's nothing radical still there. I think we got it all."

My knees sagged with relief.

Then, he added, "We won't know for sure until we do some more tests. There might still be some cancerous cells around the edge, but it will be a few days before we have the answer."

That night, Jenny and I had dinner at Philthy Phil's, where I got a little snockered and let down some of the rigid control I'd been maintaining. As we discussed the situation I found myself saying, "You know, I have to admit this is much tougher than I thought it was going to be."

She hugged me consolingly. "Don't worry, Bill...everything's going to be fine. I just know it."

Jenny was a great help in caring for her sister at home after the surgery. On the first of May, she joined Christine and I at the surgeon's office for the post-op evaluation. As we sat down with Dr. Pearlstein, we fully expected to hear that the cancer had been entirely removed and everything was fine.

Instead, he told us the cancer was still there. It was shocking news.

"What do you mean?" Christine demanded. "You cut it out, didn't you? The cancer's gone!"

"Well, we got most of it," he said slowly, "but when they tested the edges of the surrounding tissue, there were still some active cancer cells there. It was also found in your lymph nodes."

We made an appointment immediately to see the oncologist, Dr. Knipe, and returned home in a somber mood. I cradled Christine in my arms that night and we cried together, wondering where this journey was taking us.

As I held her I prayed, *Lord, please give me the strength to continue. Give me faith that although we lost this battle, we can still win the war.*

It was a bitter pill to swallow, but we still believed we were going to overcome this and that it was time to move ahead.

Two days later, on Thursday, May 3, we went to the consultation with Dr. Knipe. He said he wasn't really surprised at the results; he'd suspected some cancer would remain after surgery because of the intensity of the malignancy and the fact that it was a stage three inflammatory cancer. "This isn't the type to just go away overnight," he added.

But he was also very positive. He said that Christine had made a lot of progress, things looked good, and we were going to start a new kind of chemotherapy using a drug called Taxol. This would begin in about a week, on Thursdays. We left feeling a little brighter. Dr. Knipe felt confident about the treatment, Christine's condition had improved, and we were going forward.

Chapter 8

A COUPLE OF DAYS LATER, we attended a rather unorthodox wedding on the beach. I'd received a faxed invitation from my friend Frank, the prospective groom, a few days before the ceremony. Knowing Frank, we didn't know whether the nuptials would occur or not. We decided to show up anyway just to see what happened.

Christine wore one of the many hats she'd bought since losing her hair. Actually, she had become quite the *chapeau* collector. She had the two wigs we'd shopped for together (my favorite was still the long, blonde, Saturday Night Special). But they were hot in Florida's warm climate, and Christine spent much of her outdoor time wearing a cool and comfortable hat instead. She looked great in them, too.

The bride and groom eventually showed up, the wedding actually took place, and we went back to the newlyweds' home for a small reception. It turned out to be one of our happier days in the past few weeks. Going through chemo, enduring a radical mastectomy, then finding out the cancer was still present had delivered many blows to our confidence. But we had a great time that Saturday laughing and talking about ideas for our own wedding.

The next few days also went well. On Thursday, May 10, we returned to Chemoland. We planned these trips for Thursdays so Christine could get in a few good workdays before the worst of the side effects hit. Even though this was a new form of chemotherapy and we didn't know what to expect in the way of side effects, she was still hoping to be functional by the following Monday as she had with the other treatments.

I brought along some snacks from the health food store (I was getting to be a real pro at this), and we were greeted as old friends by the staff. They loved Christine, and said she was a good patient with a great attitude.

This new treatment didn't make Christine quite as sick, but it did make her more tired and completely sapped her energy. As she put it, "I feel like I've been hit by the Taxol truck!"

During this time, I started meditating more and occasionally attending a Buddhist center in a nearby town. That was a very peaceful period of increased introspection and prayer, and provided considerable spiritual help.

The month of May meant Devil Rays baseball, and we had a lot of fun going to the games. Christine and I usually went on Wednesday nights when Matthew, now a big boy of four, visited his father, Tom. It was good to get out for a bit, have a beer, and share some laughs. Christine was an old Toronto Blue Jays fan who really knew the game and loved it. The Devil Rays never played very well, but we still enjoyed the atmosphere.

However, Matthew needed some family fun with us, too. Just before the second bout of Christine's new and improved brand of chemo at the end of May, we took him and Mitchell, my four-year-old grandson, to Busch Gardens for the day. This was a big undertaking. Christine was up for it, though I told her if walking around and standing in line became too tiring that she should rest in the shade while I took care of the boys. First, I went on the infamous Gwazi roller coaster. Boy, was that an experience! My legs were still shaking as I walked away. The four of us went on more rides, saw many shows, and visited all the animals. Christine held up very well; the happiness and love we shared remain a treasured memory.

At the end of May, I was asked to serve as an alternate on the Development Review Board for the City of St. Pete Beach. I asked Christine if that would be a problem since this would eliminate our precious Wednesday afternoons, but my civic-minded fiancée agreed it was important that I take this job. The experience ended up being great therapy for me, as it put my mind on something new for part of the day and gave me a fresh focus. Examining cases on variances and other matters was quite interesting, and between serving on the board and all my other activities, I was quite busy.

On May 31, the Thursday following our memorable trip to Busch Gardens, Christine had her second dose of Taxol. The chemo routine had become familiar by now: bring snacks and magazines, greet the staff, read, then leave the best reading material for the next round of patients and their loved ones.

Despite her ordeal, Christine was always calm as they gave the anti-nausea medication and hooked her up to the port in her chest. Considering she was getting the crap kicked out of her on a regular basis, she was holding up well. In fact, she seemed to be getting a little better. We knew she still had cancer, but she rebounded from each treatment more quickly than the last, and her attitude was certainly more positive. Heck, by Sunday—her treatment was on Thursday—she was up for a boat trip to downtown St. Pete. She loved being on the water and out in the fresh air.

As I walked arm-in-arm with her through Straub Park, I was amazed; at this stage of her first days in chemotherapy, Christine would have been in bed and unable to eat. Instead, we were having a great day.

Chapter 9

A COUPLE OF WEEKS LATER, I figured it was high time we had some same-day fish for dinner. A friend of mine invited me to join them on an offshore fishing trip, and I had to be up and out the door by 5:00 AM. I checked on a sleepy Christine before I left to make sure she didn't need anything.

"Are you sure it's okay to go?" I asked her for the umpteenth time.

She shooed me toward the door. "Go! Have a great time!" she laughed.

Off I went. The boat was a charter, and there were six of us. We went out about twenty miles offshore and began fishing. I've had my up and down days on these trips; surprisingly, this was a good one. When we got back to shore we divided our catch, and I came home with plenty of grouper and snapper. That evening, I cooked my same-day fish for Christine,

Matthew, and me; it was incredibly delicious, if I do say so myself.

About a week later, on June 21, it was time again for Chemoland. The doctor said Christine looked good, and felt that the treatments were being effective. I talked to other people during this trip that weren't doing so well, and some who were obviously on the pathway to death. On the other hand, I met quite a few like Christine who were full of hope and confidence that they would win their individual wars.

On Friday she was tired, but Christine still felt worlds better than her earlier post-treatment days. I had registered for a week-long getaway at a retreat in Missouri called Unity Village; this was also one of the many churches that were praying for Christine. I had learned that Unity is a religion founded about a hundred years ago by Charles and Myrtle Filmore, who basically believed that we are in God's presence at all times. They also maintained that He is not a hell-and-damnation deity, but a good God who wants nothing but love, peace, and happiness for everyone. I found the concept extremely appealing, especially during this stressful time.

Arrangements for the trip had been made some time back, but I decided to wait and see how Christine was doing before confirming plans to attend. I was supposed to fly out that Saturday, two days after her treatment. We talked about it the night before. Christine insisted she was just fine and would call if necessary, but that she realized my role as caregiver was very difficult and how sorely I needed some spiritual renewal. This time it was she who held me as I cried with great relief and admitted just how right she was. The floodgates of honesty opened as I told her how hard it had been to step in and take over and what a struggle it had been. I explained earnestly that this time away in a place of quiet meditation would be the best medicine possible.

She wished me well, hugged me again, and told me to go.

The next day I went off to the airport, parked my car in the long-term lot, and boarded my flight to Kansas City, Missouri. As I stepped on the plane, I felt intuitively that something special was about to occur, and had a strongly positive vibration; while I wasn't sure just what would happen on this trip, I felt confident that it would be good.

I had a wonderful flight with no problems all the way to Kansas City, and was met at the airport by a very nice limousine driver from Unity Village's Retreat Center. The ride to Unity took almost an hour, and I spent the time looking out the window at the heartland of America in all its glory: everyday people, everyday lives, and everyone doing their thing. I thought about the situation at home and how Christine's illness had affected my life. I reflected on the additional stress, pressure, and uncertainty it had brought into my world. I also considered the fact that it had also been a period of huge personal growth.

At length, we pulled into the grounds. The minute we drove in, it was as if an aura of peace came over me: a total feeling of relaxation. Unity Village is located on about 1500 acres and includes housing for guests, two lakes, a ministerial school, and several chapels. In addition to retreats, they also offer what they call "Silent Unity," a vigil where people pray twenty-four hours a day, seven days a week. Anyone in the world can call and someone will discuss what their needs are and those people will be prayed for. It is this sort of hands-on ministry that brings such calmness to people in trauma who weren't quite sure how to deal with extreme stress; in other words, people like me.

I arrived at the housing area to check in, unpacked, then ventured outside and talked to the other folks walking around preparing themselves for the coming week. I felt an inner warmth at being in this unique part of the world where love, somehow, had become the number one priority.

Chapter 10

THE NEXT DAY, LECTURES BEGAN. These were very up-lifting and taught us about taking control of your life by con-trolling your thoughts, visualizing what you want your life to be to make it a reality, and that each one of us is captain of our own ship. I enjoyed the lectures and got to know the vari-ous participants, talked to them in the cafeteria at mealtimes, and visited a number of different chapels. A small one called the Peace Chapel was particularly appealing. There was also a large rose garden that was a great place to just sit, contemplate, and listen to your inner self. That garden became a very special place.

After a couple of days, I headed out to the lakes. It was about an hour's walk there and back, and I was looking for-ward to some exercise. There was a gently sloping gravel trail that led down through the woods, underneath an old railroad trestle, then to a fork in the road that led left to a large lake or right to a smaller one. I chose the route to the larger lake. On my left was a high railroad embankment that had been built years ago. To the right was a narrow stream that paralleled the path; its babbling music was very relaxing.

I began to get the feeling that I was being watched: as if something, somewhere was keeping an eye on me. I wasn't afraid: just a little uneasy. My trek continued over a small foot-bridge crossing the stream, then up a hill to a huge dam that held the lake in place; evidently, it had originally been much smaller. I later found out this lake provided drinking water for Unity Village. I was able to walk on top of the dam and took a look around; Dusk was approaching, there was a light breeze, and all felt beautifully peaceful. I decided this would be an ideal place to take a break and meditate.

As I sat there, a wonderful feeling of security and safety suddenly washed over me. I thought about Christine and how I had asked her to marry me on New Year's Eve. Yes, I'd already known she was a little sick before I popped the question; she was already going to the doctor for what she thought was "a little cyst."

Did she know she was more ill than she actually was and didn't tell me? I wondered. *Am I trapped? Is this some place I don't want to be, caught in her quagmire of sickness?*

I gave this a lot of deliberation before moving on to meditate further along the trail. There, I came to the realization that my true desire was to be just where I was. God had put me here, and I was evidently meant to meet this challenge and help Christine and Matthew through the crisis of cancer.

I thought about whether I felt trapped. *No,* I thought, *I could exit at any time if I wanted to. I love Christine, I love Matthew, and they're my family. Somehow, some way, we can get past all this illness, trauma, and tribulation.*

After sitting there for quite a while, I started feeling quite good as my uncertainty was erased. I now knew I was exactly where I was supposed to be.

I stood up and began the return trek to the village by a different route than the way I'd come. There was a circling path that put me on the high road above the creek in an area with many meadows. I approached a curve with a strange sense of anticipation. Rounded the corner, I saw a large meadow in which eighteen deer—yes, I counted—were grazing. The closest one was only about fifty feet away. I stopped. They lifted their heads as one to look at me. I waited for them to run, but they didn't move; we just stood there and stared at each other. I ventured a few steps closer, but they still didn't move. I was amazed. I felt that this must somehow be an extension of the peacefulness emanating from the village.

The deer closest to me seemed to be studying me closely with large, liquid eyes. He seemed to be telling me: *We don't fear you, and you're going to be all right. You have a place in this universe, just as we do, and there is nothing to be afraid of.*

As the bizarre thought occurred that a deer was talking to me by some sort of telepathy, a mist began drifting over the meadow. It just hung there and slowly enveloped all of us. The deer remained motionless and kept regarding me calmly.

That was when a voice came to me and said, "Christine is healed. Christine is well. It's all okay. Christine is healed. The sound felt like a whisper outside my body, but it didn't seem to be coming from the deer. While this was all very unsettling, I still felt a sense of peace as the voice whispered to me once more, "Christine is healed. Go...you have nothing to fear."

I stood there, totally aghast and mesmerized, not sure

whether I was dreaming this or not. Was this really happening? As I was thinking about what had just occurred, the mist lifted and wafted away as quickly as it had come. The deer turned their heads in unison and walked away across the meadow.

I watched them leave with an almost overwhelming sensation of healing, of security, of love. I began to feel warm all over, and stood there like a statue for about ten minutes.

My first step felt uncomfortable, as if I was going to fall. My uneasiness eased as I began to walk more steadily back to the village. The woods were on the right, and there were more fields on the left. As I entered a more woodsy area, I had the feeling once more that I was being watched, but it didn't concern me any more; how could anything harm me after what I'd just witnessed?

Then, I heard noises coming from the brush; it was the deer. They were actually following me back down the trail! I continued walking, hearing them moving in the bushes and catching an occasional glimpse of my four-legged companions. A couple of them popped their heads up over the bushes to the right of me, a few more then to my far right. Frankly, things were beginning to get a little spooky again.

But the eerie feeling was abruptly replaced by the sense that God was there, and that He or one of His guardian angels was looking over my shoulder to make sure I was okay. For some reason, He had come to tell me that Christine was going to be well. And the deer? They seemed to be escorting me back because they could sense I was extremely wobbly. They were right. My feet felt like mush, and my legs were like spaghetti as I slowly walked back to my room. I reached the little footbridge where I'd crossed the creek before, then went under a tunnel underneath the railroad trestle and up a hill through the woods.

I had the sudden urge to turn around. There they were: two deer in the trail behind me. They were a hundred feet away at the most. After a few moments, they turned and walked back down the trail toward the woods. It was as if they were telling me, *we got you back, and you're safe. You can go home now.*

I covered the short distance back to my room feeling as if I'd just run the Boston Marathon. Once there, I undressed and lay in bed with a total feeling of awe until I fell into a deep sleep that was full of restfulness and healing.

The next day, I woke up feeling as if a huge weight had been lifted from my shoulders. I knew that on that walk God had told me that everything was going to be okay, and that the pressure of Christine's illness and the problems surrounding it were now solved. I lay in bed for a while, thinking about what had happened out there in the woods with the deer and the mist and the voice, musing about this mystical experience in a mystical forest. I smiled. God was truly here at Unity Village, and He had let me know it was going to be okay. I didn't feel particularly special; I was just one among many here looking for help, a solution, a cure. I was here because I loved Christine, and wanted to see Matthew's little face smiling if Mommy got better.

I got dressed, and went to the Peace Chapel after breakfast. There were plenty of places to pray at Unity Village, but I felt especially comfortable there. It was a small building, with only about six or eight seats. It also had a little slot to submit a prayer request form. I filled out a form and asked Unity to pray for Christine and help heal her cancer, then added a donation.

As I dropped the envelope into the little slot, the voice I had heard in the woods said clearly in a soft, comforting tone, "Your prayers are already answered. It's taken care of."

I sat down in one of the chairs to pray about it all. The same warmth crept over me that I had experienced in the woods of comfort, relaxation, and total peace.

As I gloried in this sense of Divine love, the voice spoke once more. "I told you last night, everything is okay. Everything is going to be fine, and Christine is healed," it said. "She is healed."

Chapter 11

AFTER ABOUT AN HOUR, I departed feeling totally uplifted and filled with an intense, joyful certainty that a divine healing had somehow taken place. I walked slowly back to my motel room to call Christine. When I got her voice mail instead, I left a message that I was thinking about her, and that I knew from what had happened here at Unity Village that everything was going to be okay. I didn't say any more than that; what had happened in the woods was weird enough for me to acknowledge, let alone telling someone else about it...even Christine.

I thoroughly enjoyed the quiet peacefulness during the last few days of my retreat, and even played golf (on top of everything else, they had a nine-hole course). I shot in the upper 80s for two times around, which is very good for me.

I returned to the Peace Chapel to pray and meditate just before my departure. I gave thanks for this mystical place and the presence of God that had intervened for my beloved and me. He had indeed done what a loving God would do, and there is no question in my mind that The Lord does live in Unity Village.

I thought about the Silent Unity Chapel nearby, where people prayed for everyone who had submitted requests, including mine and Christine's. *They're doing such wonderful work for people in need all over the world*, I thought. *But what about people who don't believe in God? What about those who don't have Him to turn to? That is really sad…and disappointing.* I felt incredible sympathy for those unfortunate folks. Truly, I had God to turn to—and in regard to Christine's illness, He had come through with flying colors. It is wonderful to know that when things are troubling me, I can always turn to the Lord and Unity for help.

I walked out of the chapel toward the waiting limousine. As it headed out of the village, I looked over my shoulder. *Wow, now I have to go back to the real world. I have to go back to the place where love isn't always number one on everyone's list… where love of power overshadows the power of love.* I sighed as my safe haven receded into the distance.

I reached the airport with mixed feelings. While happy to be going home to Christine and Matthew, there was also sadness at leaving Unity Village and its atmosphere of rest, comfort, and peace. But happiness won out; I now knew my fiancée was healed, and that it was time to talk about getting married. My flight arrived at Tampa International Airport late in the evening. I picked up my car and drove home leisurely, serene in the assurance that all was well with Christine.

The following morning was Saturday and I awakened relaxed, as if a heavy weight had been taken off my shoulders. I lay there thinking about what had occurred during the past few days. *What mystical experience had I been part of? Should I say anything to Christine?* I weighed the possible consequences. *If everything I was told is true, then she is healed. On the other hand, if I tell her what happened and it turns out not to be true, there will be tremendous disappointment.* I decided not to mention any specifics about the trip: just that it had been a positive experience.

I got up and dressed. My son Erik and his wife Amanda were expecting a little girl in less than a month, and this was the day Christine and I were going shopping for a baby shower gift. We bought a truly ingenious stroller that converted into a car seat and baby tote. The following day, Sunday, July 1, our family celebrated this new life about to come into the world. I smiled at my inner conviction that Christine's life was also a celebration that was going to continue.

Chapter 12

ON JULY 12, IT WAS time for another excursion to Chemoland. I brought along gifts and little treats for the nurses: cookies and other goodies the staff and visitors really enjoyed. Christine and I talked to people and read magazines while she received her treatment. As was usual toward the end of these sessions, she became quite tired and sat back in her lounge chair with her eyes closed. I sat there watching her face and thinking about what had happened at Unity Village. I wanted to tell her so badly about my experience, but was afraid that if anything went wrong it would be a huge letdown. Although I firmly believed the voice that told me she'd been healed, I decided once more to just shut my mouth and keep on praying.

Christine ended up walking out of there after a while feeling pretty well; the doctor had told her she was making excellent progress, and she was looking better, too. By Saturday her condition had improved so much that that I proposed a trip down to Sanibel-Captiva Island. We drove down to a resort called Tweenwaters where we had a fabulous dinner, then danced to the live band in the bar. As I held my fiancée in my arms, I recalled the many times early in her treatment that people we knew greeted us and the minute Christine's back was turned, they asked me if she was going to die. This weekend, things were different. I detected a spark in her eyes I hadn't seen in a long time.

I was impressed anew by this seemingly fragile woman's strength. As much as she had been knocked out by the many treatments she'd undergone, she had kept her head above water and continued to work. Many patients we'd met at Chemoland didn't work at all during their treatment. Christine, on the other hand, managed to run a realty office of about thirty people who were all very supportive of their boss. Such a positive atmosphere was good for her self-esteem, and I admired her determination to keep working.

We went to my grandson Mitchell's fifth birthday party the following week. Matthew had a ball playing with the birthday boy, and it was a festive evening. Again, I saw a glimpse of the healthy Christine I had known. I was further convinced when she signed us up to participate in the Realtor's Political Action Committee bowling fundraiser the following Saturday. This was an extracurricular activity she could easily have bowed out of, but she insisted on being part of her crew, and they were thrilled to see her. What would have devastated Christine physically just weeks ago turned out to be a fun and exhilarating afternoon.

During this progressively recuperative period, I became concerned about Matthew and Mitchell's swimming abilities; after all, we were surrounded by water on Florida's Gulf

Coast and so many of our friends and neighbors had swimming pools. I signed them up for a course offered by the local park service at 6:00 PM on Tuesdays and Thursdays, and drove them to each hour-long lesson. I was pleased and proud at the boys' rapid progress into tadpoles, and it was especially fun when Christine's schedule permitted her to join us. It also got Matthew over the fear of putting his head under water. He was soon jumping into the pool from the deep end.

Shortly after Christine's last chemotherapy treatment we went to see Dr. Knipe, who reported that all Christine's test results were good.

"I think we're ready to begin radiation treatment," he announced.

Christine and I looked at each other. We'd both done our homework, and already knew this other side of the cancer treatment coin was decidedly unpleasant. While chemotherapy assaulted the disease internally, radiation was intended to literally burn the cancer away from the outside. I saw Christine take a deep breath as Dr. Knipe explained that the radiation would focus on four strategic locations. We were told that though most people have the radiation focused on only one area, the fact that her cancer had spread to the lymph nodes made this more aggressive approach necessary. The treatment would take place Monday through Friday for seven weeks.

The radiologist, Dr. Franzese, explained that the sickness from the chemotherapy was different from that of radiation. The skin became very burned and crispy-looking, and it was necessary to use a lot of moisturizer to control the damage.

Dr. Franzese was clearly not one to mince words. "To put it quite simply, Christine," he added graphically, "after seven weeks of treatment, you will appear very much like a burn victim."

Our trip from Chemoland to Radiationland was a short one; the facility was almost directly across the street, and operated like an outpatient area of the hospital. I went to the first couple of sessions with Christine in case there were any problems, but she quickly got used to the sensation of burning and seemed fully capable of driving afterward. She seemed to deal with it well, though it was hard for me to watch her skin darkening and drying so rapidly.

Toward the end of the month—July 27, to be exact—joy came into our lives in the form of Haley, Erik and Amanda's new baby girl. She was an utterly healthy, gorgeous expression of life, and her birth was an affirming experience for us all. It was a nice change to be around the hospital for a happier occasion than cancer treatment. Our new granddaughter made us both very happy.

August came. The radiologist explained that as the radiation continued, Christine could expect to feel worse than she was feeling now, and that things would get a little rougher. He hastened to add that she was "doing great."

I was spending some time at Erik's house because of Haley's arrival. Mitchell was starting to get a little jealous over all the attention his baby sister was getting, and I figured I could use a little break from the recent impact of Christine's treatments. She and I agreed that it would be a good idea if I took Mitchell to Chicago for a long weekend. He could visit his grandmother, aunts, and uncles, and it would assure him that he was still very special.

I rented a car when we landed in the Windy City and drove to my brother Jim's house. After getting Mitchell settled, Jim and his wife, Trish, babysat while I went out with my other brother Ed and his friends to a White Sox game. It was like a trip back to my childhood, getting on a bus with forty people and taking off for the ballpark. There was also a keg of beer, which added greatly to the festivities. I spent the night at Ed's house and headed back to Jim's the next morning, where Mitchell was quite happy to see me.

We also celebrated Jim's birthday. My mother, Mitchell's great-grandmother, really loved having all of her boys together, and showered Mitchell with all the attention any child could wish for. We picked up Mom the following day and took her to lunch at an excellent restaurant before heading to the airport. This relaxing five days had done me a world of good, and Mitchell seemed to approach his sister's arrival a little more gracefully.

When we got home, I found that Christine's reaction to the radiation was getting worse, just as Dr. Franzese had predicted. But on August 11, she showed her true colors again. The Kiwanis Club, of which I was a member, was having their annual Care Fair at a local middle school. This is a major event attended by thousands of disadvantaged children in the community whose parents can't afford school physicals or supplies. I was in charge of V.I.P. parking, which involved waving cars in and out and keeping track of local television crews. Christine insisted on coming to help, only asking that her job be inside where she could sit down. She found a perfect spot at check-in, helping families become organized and get immunization shots for their kids.

My friend Kathy was running the Care Fair. " It's just fabulous that Christine can help under her circumstances," she marveled.

I smiled and agreed; this was all just business-as-usual for my remarkable wife-to-be. Christine worked all day. When we had lunch together, the twinkle in her eyes somehow reminded me of my surreal encounter at Unity Village.

God put that look there, I thought. It was hard not to share my profound experience with her, but instinct still told me to remain silent.

The morning after the Care Fair I thought Christine would be exhausted, but she seemed to be in great spirits. There must be something about the vibration we receive when helping others instead of concentrating on ourselves; instead of tiring us, it makes us stronger. We went to church in the morning, then returned that afternoon for a seminar. During this full day of devotion I thanked God for the healing He had done during what I now thought of as the "mysticism in the village."

Chapter 13

THE FOLLOWING WEEK, WE WENT boating for the day to Shell Island. Matthew had a great time chasing crabs and watching fish in the clear water. It was good to feel the warmth of the sun and the loving power of nature holding us, healing us.

September 4 was my birthday, and it was time for a barbecue. Erik came over with Amanda, Mitchell, and Haley, who was now a little over a month old. A few other close friends joined us, I grilled big slabs of salmon, and had a wonderful birthday that made becoming a year older quite bearable. My best gift was seeing Christine holding up so well and thoroughly enjoying herself.

The radiation burns were getting quite intense for her by now, and she was always applying lotion. She looked like she'd been badly burned in a fire. I was spending a lot of time giving massages and holding her in reassurance and support. We were near the end of treatment when the effects became the worst, and it was quite a tough go of it. But Christine kept her head up and pushed on; she knew she was beating this thing.

The weekend after Labor Day, we went out for dinner at the Bonefish Grill, then to a concert at church. It was very peaceful and beautiful. I felt a warm feeling of God all about us.

The next day, Saturday, we went north and stayed in a small Florida town named Micanopy. There's an old attraction called the Herlong mansion that is reportedly haunted by a former resident. We didn't stay in the mansion itself but in the carriage house, which had been converted into an efficiency apartment with a hot tub. It was a great place to stay, and we didn't see any ghosts.

We attended a game that night at Gainesville's University of Florida, and watched their Gators win in "The Swamp," which is what they appropriately call their stadium.

They had bikes at the mansion, which we rode into town to visit the ice cream parlor. It was like being kids again, riding bikes and eating ice cream cones. Christine and I had quite a romantic interlude, despite her burns.

The next week was just horrible. On September 11, 2001, the world seemed to stand still as two planes flew into New York's World Trade Center. I was at home working when Christine called and told me to turn on the television. I sat there stunned, watching the horrific events unfold: people jumping out of the doomed towers, thousands more crushed to death under tons of rubble…it was all too sad to comprehend. There were no words to describe the tragedy.

Our nation was upset and saddened—and it wanted revenge. It was hard to stay positive, and combined with our battle against Christine's cancer, we were both knocked a little off-center by this world's earth-shaking events for a while.

It was only a few days after the attack that Christine finished her final round of radiation treatments. The doctor told her all the reports were good, and the oncologist said that all her tests looked excellent. In other words, the cancer was gone.

We decided that in view of this, it was time for a weekend getaway to the Florida Keys. On Friday, September 21, we took off to Key Largo to celebrate "the end of the burning." Christine's skin was still very crispy and while the salt water was very good for healing, it also stung her like crazy when we went snorkeling. She stood it for as long as she could, but after a few hours she wanted to head back to the condo we'd rented and shower off the painful salt.

We were booked for a four-day weekend and it was obvious Christine couldn't go in the water any more, so we took a fishing charter instead. We were the only ones signed up, and a husband and wife guide team took us on a quest for mahi-mahi. I was used to cruising the Gulf of Mexico along St. Petersburg Beach, but being in the Keys meant we were basically fishing in the Atlantic Ocean and were able to get to deep water much more quickly. I can still see the huge smile on Christine's face when she hooked her first big one: a beautiful, deep blue mahi that she brought up to the boat without help. She was quite proud of herself, and I was proud of her, too.

We caught quite a few fish that afternoon, and being out at sea was good for Christine. All the activity was still a little rough on her, but she handled the physical stress well and enjoyed fishing. I could see life vibrating all about her, and the aura of impending doom seemed to have lifted. That's what our existence was all about: feeling life, enjoying life, being a part of life; knowing that life just *is*.

We were a bit tired when we finally docked the boat, so we decided to relax for the rest of the day with some shopping. That was the day we found "Jake," a wooden dolphin statue. Jake now greets people when they come to our front door, and has become a part of our family. Our cat, Eliza, enjoys rubbing up against him tremendously.

After we returned to St. Pete Beach and home, Christine discovered her co-workers had organized a party at one of their homes to honor her fortieth birthday. It was quite a blast, with great drinks and unbelievable food, including stuffed mushrooms and shrimp. It was a perfect Florida evening with a cool sea breeze, and a very happy birthday for Christine.

The following Sunday, September 30, little Haley was to be christened at Pasadena Church. My daughter, Kellie, arrived from California to serve as godmother. We had a family get-together at Erik and Amanda's house afterward. Christine was there and feeling pretty good, and Matthew was joyfully playing with my grandson Mitchell. The welcoming of Haley into the Christian community was a wonderful family event.

Another such joyful event was Matthew's fifth birthday on Monday, when we had a party at Chuckie Cheese with a number of his friends. Erik, Amanda, and Kellie were there with Haley, and we all played lots of games with Mitchell, Matthew, and the other kids. It was an exciting time and a real boost of childhood energy for the adults. I looked over at Christine and saw the huge smile on her face, noting that her color was better than it had been in a while.

The following Friday, my good friend Dimitri flew in from Colorado. We picked him up at the airport, reunited him with my family, then all took off for Bern's Steak House, one of the finest in the country and a place the President likes to dine whenever he is in town. Here you buy your steak by weight as well as the cut. We celebrated Christine and Kellie's birthdays and had a fine time. After dinner, the staff gave us a tour of the kitchen to show us how everything was made before making our way upstairs to the restaurant's famed Dessert Room. We sat and enjoyed our desserts in comfort, complete with our own jukebox. The desserts were decadent, chocolate indulgences that were simply heavenly.

Dimitri took me aside. "You know, Bill, Christine looks a little more chipper than she did on my last visit."

"She does, doesn't she?" I beamed. "She's really getting better."

We went to breakfast on the beach the next morning. My friend Gary Wapinski was in town, and joined us along with Erik, Amanda, Dimitri, and Kellie. Christine was busy getting packed for our upcoming trip to Canada. Kellie was going to be leaving for California later that day, at almost the same time we'd be flying with Matthew to Canada to see Christine's family for Canadian Thanksgiving, which is observed on a different day than in America.

After enjoying a great breakfast while watching the waves roll in, we went our separate ways: Kellie back to sunny California; Christine, Matthew and I to the Great White North. We arrived very late that night in Halifax, rented a car at the airport and drove for about an hour to Christine's sister Jenny's house. Jenny and her husband Rob, their daughter Leah, and Christine's mother, Marilyn, were overjoyed to see her. It was a touching reunion. We spent Sunday relaxing and exploring the beautiful Nova Scotia countryside.

The following day, Monday, was Thanksgiving. We had a huge feast, and the family was thrilled to see that Christine was doing a bit better. She didn't have much hair yet, but you could tell it was starting to grow back. We all gave thanks and celebrated a brighter future facing the wonderful woman we all love.

The following day, Christine and I headed off to Cape Breton. We stayed at a place called the Celtic Lodge that jutted out into the Atlantic: a rustic, fascinating place with a distinguished history. We dined the first night in the very elegant dining room among very elegant-looking people.

The next day we went back to Jenny's with a bunch of live lobsters and had great fun chasing them around the kitchen. Once they were off the floor and on our plates where they belonged, the result was absolutely delicious.

Before we knew it, the week was up and it was time to leave. On the 13th, we flew back to St. Petersburg and resumed our normal activities. This included getting an important belated birthday gift for Matthew. We had promised him a kitten from one of Christine's friends who had a surplus of felines, and had given him all the necessary equipment for responsible cat ownership: a kitty bed, food, a litter box, and so on. It was now time to pick up Eliza (Matthew had already chosen the name). We took her to the vet, then home to become the newest member of our family. With Christine's illness looming in the background and the long process of healing, this new family member was a joy that brought lots of smiles and happiness to our home.

We decided it was time for a little inspiration and went to a lecture by renowned author Wayne Dyer, who was appearing in person at St. Petersburg's Mahaffey Theater. It was great to feel reaffirmed that we all have the power to heal, and that illness doesn't have to own us. I recaptured that good feeling I had experienced at Unity Village, and emerged with renewed conviction that the words I had heard at Unity were words of truth.

This truly was a world where we were captains of our own ships, and had the power within ourselves to lead a life filled with good health and prosperity.

Chapter 14

SHORTLY AFTER THE WAYNE DYER talk, we had an appointment with the radiologist. He looked at the test results and told us that everything still looked good, and there were no signs of any new cancer. This was fabulous news. True, the burns were still deep and painful, but were visibly healing.

Christine and I decided that we were up to watching Haley and Mitchell so that Erik and Amanda could have an evening free. The following Saturday we took them along with Matthew to Circus McGirkus in St. Pete, which might best be described as an annual peace festival. There were social justice booths, the Sierra Club, Greenpeace, church promotions, and a lot of tie-dyed clothes and talks about world peace. It was a positive place to spend the afternoon, and the kids had a great time.

Speaking of social awareness, Christine participated just a

week later in the Tampa Bay Heart Walk, in which her company was actively involved. The Heart Walk was taking place in Tampa, near the Ice Palace where the Tampa Bay Lightning Hockey Team plays. Christine and I joined a number of her co-workers and had a great time walking, campaigning, and celebrating for the good of humankind. The same evening, we also attended a Sierra Club fundraising dinner at Sunken Gardens in St. Petersburg.

November 8 was a special occasion. Christine had grown a little hair by this point. It still looked rather like a crewcut, but it was *hair*. We had a photo taken with Matthew for our family portrait. The three of us had dinner out afterward and she was in great spirits, though she was to have surgery the next day. First, the doctors were taking the port out, since they didn't think she was going to need any more chemotherapy. They were also going to remove her ovaries as a precaution; the doctors felt it was wise to remove a target area where cancer could very possibly pop up.

The following morning, I took Matthew to school and went on to the hospital. This surgery promised to be an interesting procedure, since it would give them a chance to go in and take a look around. I remember sitting there waiting for the surgeon to come out; he sat down with me and announced that everything had gone smoothly, Christine was in Recovery, and there was no signs of cancer anywhere.

Thank you, God, I prayed silently.

The doctor added that they would continue to watch her for a few months, but that everything looked very good indeed. "After that," he said with a smile, "we can begin to look at reconstruction."

We had definitely turned the corner. Through her desire to live and God's grace, Christine was healed...just as the voice had told me at Unity Village. All she had to do now was re-cover, get strong, and eventually, they would begin the process of putting her back together.

It was just a week later when two well-known business people from the St. Pete Beach community invited me out to lunch. They wanted to discuss the upcoming city elections, and said that the positions of mayor and a spot on the city council were open. They also told me that I had a lot of support, and they would like me to consider running for city council. I told them Christine had more tests coming up within the next month; I would have to wait to discuss it with her and get back to them. It was interesting to see their desire for me to represent the people of the community, and I considered it at the very least a pat on the back.

As one of the trustee members of the Brightwater-Punta Vista Association, I took an opportunity at their annual block party the next Saturday to discuss the possibility of running for city council. Everyone was very positive about the idea and suggested I pursue it.

Flattering though this was, I had plenty of other work to keep my feet on the ground. I had become involved with a newspaper recycling center that hired the disadvantaged. Some of the people were mildly handicapped, and the center was a little behind in production. A few of my fellow Kiwanis Club members joined me to help by standing inside huge bins filled with paper and feeding the contents onto conveyor belts, which dumped the load in the bailer. It made for an interesting evening.

In mid-December, we decided to move our company, Allard Investment Realty, from its current suite to another in the same building. The move was from an upstairs location to a slightly smaller one downstairs, which would be more compact and save a few dollars on rent. It was also a more advantageous position. The stressful process was soon accomplished.

During the move Christine had more tests that all showed everything was still fine. However, the doctors still wanted to wait a few more months to let her skin heal before they considered reconstructive surgery.

On Saturday, December 15, we decided to take a canoe trip weekend on the Withlacoochee River. While drifting through the water, we celebrated Christine's test results and discussed the possibility of my running for city council. There were a lot of issues dividing people in our community, and Christine said she felt I would stand up and speak out about what was right and wrong without fear of ridicule. I decided to file the papers to run for election the next month.

We also discussed the topic of our wedding and setting a date. Christine made it very clear to me that she wanted to have hair and her breasts reconstructed before walking down the aisle. She said her doctors told her that reconstruction would take place in the coming year, but it might take that long until everything was completed.

"It's important for me to feel whole, Bill," she said simply.

I understood completely, and we agreed that the following year would be a better time. If all went well, we would get married in February of 2003.

Delay or not, it was great to be making wedding plans at last.

Chapter 15

THE WEEK FOLLOWING THE CANOE trip, deceit reared its ugly head in our home community. A group tried to sneak through increases on building heights and densities by scheduling a meeting just a week before Christmas. They'd obviously calculated that everyone would be busy with holiday shopping and anticipated there would be few, if any, voices of dissension. I made it my business to make sure word got out, and on the appointed day we were able to defeat the measure and have the issue tabled for the next few months. It was a good feeling to handle this on a grassroots level with my fellow citizens.

That Friday, December 21, was our Allard Investment Realty Christmas party. We had a great time at the Vinoy Resort, a beautiful Mediterranean-style villa on Tampa Bay. We enjoyed a jazz band and great food while celebrating the end of a horrific year and the hopeful beginning of a better one. It was great to see Christine showing her inner vitality once again, and everyone had a ball.

On the 27th, my daughter Kellie arrived in town for a belated Christmas dinner and celebration at Erik and Amanda's house. During this holiday visit Christine and I took Kellie out on the boat with Dimitri. Things got very exciting at one point when some large waves threatened to capsize us, but we were able to get back into safe waters, thank God. It was truly an experience that had all of us holding our collective breath.

New Year's Eve, 2001: I took Kellie to the airport and she headed back to California. Christine and I went out to dinner and a hockey game with some friends, then on to Dimitri's new house for champagne. My friend had finally moved to Florida.

There was a moment when he and I looked at each other, knowing we were thinking the same thing. It was hard to believe that only a year ago we were standing in a dark parking lot as I showed Dimitri Christine's diamond ring and told him I was about to propose. We were almost overwhelmed by what the last year had been, and the journey we had taken. What sacrifices had been made! But now, Christine was almost well again.

Thank you, God, I prayed silently.

Dimitri smiled and raised his glass to me in an understanding salute.

On January 1, 2002, we began Christine's year of reconstruction by going to her friend Jeanne's for a wonderful lunch, then to dinner that night at another friend's home. Christine was feeling more social, and we were getting more and more invitations. I was still a bit apprehensive about her condition;

after all, for months she had lived on the edge of death. While she was looking forward to her reconstruction, I felt as if I was holding my breath to see if any cancer was going to recur.

On January 2, I picked up the election package from City Hall and sat down to go over it with Christine, who was very supportive. I filled out the paperwork, got the necessary signatures, and filed to run for city council in the March election. I began attending council meetings and hearing about the issues. One major furor involved building a new city hall for four million dollars without bidding it out. Instead, the job had been given to a well-known "friend" of the council. In reviewing the cost incurred, it was obvious the city could have done much better if competitive bids had been taken. Another idea the council was pushing was to increase building heights from a maximum of 50 to 100 feet, which the community didn't like at all. Though I found the deception of politics disheartening, I pursued my campaign and recruited volunteers, donations, and helpers.

I also spent some time with my little brother from the Big Brothers/Big Sisters program. Kenny was a senior in high school now, and doing just great. I'd gone to see him play basketball—he scored 28 points that night, and broke the school season record for most points over 1,000.

Keith, his brother, was back in school and also doing well. He was getting his grades up in hopes that next year he would be academically eligible to play, too. I took them both on as little brothers when they were 9 and 10 years old, and realized after about three meetings that they couldn't read. I purchased the Hooked on Phonics program, the family became involved, and the boys began doing much better. In fact, Kenny was now looking at a college basketball scholarship.

I had my first election debate on February 13. It was quite

a rude awakening for me in the political arena. I realized that my opponents were lying outright, and spent time researching data after the debate to prove it. But when I showed my prospective constituents the truth, much to my surprise they just shook their heads and said resignedly, "Well, they're politicians, aren't they? They *all* lie."

I guess the thought that I might not be successful in politics first occurred to me at that debate. The opposition blithely told people what they wanted to hear without any facts or figures to back it up, and I simply couldn't live with lying to my community.

On Saturday, February 23, Christine's sister, Jenny, arrived from Canada for a visit. On the night she arrived, we took her to Clearwater for a party at our friend Anton's house. Dimitri came along, too. Anton passed out some expensive Cuban cigars as a special treat, and we all had a terrific time.

One of the reasons Jenny had come to Florida was to go with us to the reconstruction doctor, Dr. Rehnke, the following Tuesday. We had a good meeting in which he checked Christine over completely and announced that he could definitely help.

"You're doing well," he told her, "but you're not quite healed enough to begin reconstruction."

One breast had been completely removed in the first mastectomy; the other had smaller amounts of cancer and had remained. Removing it as a precaution and rebuilding both was now being considered. It was going to be quite a medical project, to say the least, and Dr. Rehnke wanted to wait a few months to make very sure no new cancer reappeared.

"If all goes well, perhaps we can begin in May," he told us.

He smiled gently at my fiancée's crestfallen expression. "Don't worry, Christine…we'll get there."

She was frustrated by the delay, but consoled herself that we had at least the possibility of a target date.

Chapter 16

LATER THAT WEEK, JENNY LEFT for Canada. It had been a great visit that had helped us all no end, and we were sorry to see her go. On Friday, March 1, we took a break from the campaign and everything else to go to the Plant City Strawberry Festival. This annual event is well known for country exhibits, great rides, and, of course, strawberries. Matthew really enjoyed all the rides on the midway, and we all ate our fill of strawberry shortcake with whipped cream. To top it all off, we saw the Charlie Daniels Band that night at the fairgrounds. Even five-year-old Matthew enjoyed the music, and we all had a fabulous time.

The following week brought a lot of campaigning; the election was coming up fast. On March 7, I appeared in a televised debate with the other candidates. I spent a lot time pointing out lies I had discovered, and backed them up with concrete facts and figures. My aggravation mounted as I saw these liars smiling blandly into the camera as if I was discussing the weather. Perhaps because of my frustration, I felt I didn't come across very well to the audience.

The election was March 12. We got up early and went down to the polls to help out and talk to my constituents. No one received more than fifty percent of the vote in the final tally, so the top two candidates—the incumbent and me—were slated for a runoff on April 2.

Exhausted from campaigning and badly in need of a break, we left on March 14 for San Francisco and Lake Tahoe to visit my daughter, Kellie. Matthew stayed with his father this time. We skied, gambled in the casino, relaxed in the spas, dined in great restaurants, and generally had some badly needed, all-adult fun. When Kellie had to return to work after a very enjoyable weekend, Christine and I took off for Calestoga in the Napa Valley. We stayed at a spa there and got massaged, took mud baths, and generally took advantage of this time to be pampered.

We returned to Florida in great shape on March 20. We still had two weeks until the runoff election, and the Allard for City Council campaigners knocked on neighborhood doors with renewed energy. I talked to many people about the way their local officials were cheating them, and found many receptive ears, On April 2, the runoff was held. We won at the polls but lost the absentee ballots, so the incumbent won by 15 votes.

We had a party at our home that evening to thank all our hard-working volunteers, and it was a celebration despite the loss. Looking back on the entire experience now, I think perhaps I wasn't meant for politics. While I enjoyed talking to people and having an active role in city government, dealing with some of the area's movers and shakers made me feel as if I was looking under rocks for vermin.

A couple of my friends saw me a week after the election and said, "Bill, you're just not a good liar. Unfortunately, lying well is what you need to do to be a politician."

I shrugged and replied, "Well, that's just not going to influence my character. Lying has never been my cup of tea, and I'm certainly not going to start now just to get people to vote for me."

And that was my big adventure into the world of politics. Did I miss the attention? The campaigning? Like any logical human being, I'd rather go fishing instead. So on Saturday, April 6, I took Christine out for her first backwater guided excursion. We won the trip at a charity auction, and the prospect of a half-day on the water with an expert was an exciting one. It was evident from the way she handled herself that afternoon that she was getting stronger every day...and it was great for both of us to get back to a "normal" life after the election.

Chapter 17

ONE OF THE UPCOMING JOYS of our lives was the formal celebration of Erik and Amanda's wedding, a very elegant social event scheduled for Saturday, April 27. The far more casual shower was held on April 7 at Fort Desoto Park, a lovely beach with a historic Spanish fort that was quite a tourist attraction.

Everyone had a blast riding Erik and Amanda's Jet Skis and enjoying great food. I could sense our younger guests, Matthew and Mitchell, were getting a bit impatient with boring grownup festivities, so I took them on a walk to investigate the fort. They really enjoyed running around to check out the old cannons and delightfully creepy jail cells.

The beautiful, breezy Sunday afternoon was a perfect day for an outdoor celebration, and Christine and I enjoyed ourselves as a couple in love.

On Thursday, April 11, I had to go to a mediation hearing regarding real estate earnest money in Fort Lauderdale. I got up early for the four-hour drive, handled the hearing successfully, then headed to Boca Raton to meet my friend, Barry, for a couple of days of relaxation and fishing. After a great dinner at a local restaurant, we were heading for the door when Barry tripped and fell...hard. I turned to see him lying on the ground with blood pouring from a head wound. I rushed to call an ambulance, called his wife, picked her up, and we rushed to the emergency room. My friend had taken quite a traumatic hit to the head, and it was three in the morning before I got his wife back to their house.

When I got to the hospital the next day, Barry looked like he'd run into a Mack truck. They kept him there for a week, but it seemed he would be all right.

I couldn't help but think that I was somehow fated to be involved with hospitals; I'd spent countless hours in them with Christine, and now here I was with Barry, surrounded by the all-too familiar antiseptic smells and white-coated personnel. I ended up coming back to St. Pete on Friday night and fell into bed, exhausted.

I had recovered sufficiently by the next Saturday when CASA, a charity organization, held a black tie dinner and silent auction to raise money for assisting spouse and child victims of domestic violence. Christine and I dressed to the nines and had a great time bidding at the auction and as luck would have it, we won a wedding package with a local videographer. We made arrangements to use his services at our wedding the following February. We chose February 15 because it was the Saturday closest to Valentine's Day, an astrologer we knew had suggested it, and Christine had made it quite clear that she was not walking down the aisle until all the surgeries were over and she was looking and feeling her best.

Wednesday, the 24th, the guests began arriving for Erik and Amanda's wedding. I played hooky from work and took my brother Joe, his wife, and Matthew fishing. My mother arrived that evening and came to my house for dinner, along with my other brother Ed and his wife. We cooked, talked, and had a wonderful family get-together in anticipation of this very happy occasion. My daughter Kellie arrived the next day, and we booked her into the hotel on the beach where Mom was staying. That Friday was the rehearsal dinner—or, in this case, a lakeside picnic with family and friends. We rented a canoe and glided around the lake, enjoying the scenery and the warmth of having our loved ones all together.

Saturday was the big day. The gentlemen of the wedding party started the morning with a few rounds of golf, which was enjoyed by all (regardless of the score). That evening I stood up as best man for my son, and no father could have been prouder. Amanda was beautiful, as was the ceremony at the Sanibel Harbor Resort. The room Erik and Amanda hired had a glorious view of the water and the reception went off without a hitch; truly the stuff from which fairy tales are made.

One mental image that will stay with me for a lifetime is that of my brother Eddie doing the Pogo at the wedding. He caused quite a stir on the dance floor. While I'm sure I'm not the only one who will remember it, perhaps Eddie wishes we would all forget.

Christine and I picked up Mitchell and baby Haley the next day for a nine-day stay with us while Erik and Amanda honeymooned in Europe, proving that there is virtually nothing parents won't do for their children. The day after the happy couple left, Christine and I took my mom, Kellie, my brother

Jim, his fiancée Trish, and the grandkids boating for the day. Mom left for Chicago and Kellie for San Francisco the next day, Mitchell returned to school, and Haley spent the day with me. She wasn't quite a year old yet, and it was nice to know my parenting skills hadn't gotten too rusty. By the weekend we decided on another boating trip, so Christine, Mitchell, Matthew, Haley, and I went out for the day. Christine was feeling strong and doing well, and spending the day with the children was a joy.

When Erik and Amanda returned from a glorious honeymoon, we handed over the children with smiles of happy exhaustion. The timing was good, because the day after that Jenny came back to town to help me support her sister through the surgery. All in all, having the kids for a prolonged stay had helped keep Christine's mind off the operation and focused on positive things.

We got up at the crack of dawn on May 8 and headed for the hospital. There would be a total mastectomy of the remaining breast, and reconstructive surgery on the side heavily damaged by radiation. It was a nine-hour procedure with two surgeons, and the lengthy anxiety was extremely hard on those of us in the waiting room. It was difficult to think of Christine spending so much time under the knife.

Jenny and I had to wait a few hours until the surgeon who had done the mastectomy came out to have a word with us. My first question was whether they'd found any new cancerous tissue. He said all had gone well, and that while he wouldn't be certain until the lab tests came back, he was relatively confident that there was no new cancer apparent.

After the mastectomy was complete, it was time for Dr. Rehnke, the reconstructive surgeon, to step up to the plate. After ten hours had passed since they wheeled Christine into the

OR, he emerged looking very worn out, and sat down to talk to me and Jenny. He explained that the procedure had taken longer than anticipated because the area had been irradiated from four different locations, and the skin was so damaged that it was extremely difficult to work with. However, he was finally able to place everything where it should be and all was well. It would be a while before she woke up—perhaps even the next day—but she was going to be just fine.

Jenny and I left the hospital with tearful relief and decided to get a bite to eat at a nearby Italian restaurant. When we got back, Christine was semiconscious. We talked to her reassuringly, and she occasionally opened an eye in acknowledgement, but it was quite clear she was still under the effects of the anesthesia. The nurses suggested that we go home to rest and come back the next day.

Jenny and I went home, had a couple of cocktails to blow off some steam, and went to the club down the street to unwind a bit. We talked a lot about Christine, the surgery, and life in general, and I realized anew just how very stressful all this was. It was a lot like our conversation some months ago when this ordeal began, and Jenny was very supportive. I realized I was doing much better than I had been back then; I was much more realistic now about how much the cancer trauma had knocked me on my ass.

After a good night's sleep, Jenny and I went for a walk on the beach before going to the hospital.

We faced a groggy but smiling Christine. "I want to go home," she said distinctly.

Unfortunately, the hospital staff wasn't quite so sure, and it wasn't until late afternoon that they finally released her. Jenny and I got the newly remodeled Christine into the car and home to recover in her own bed. What a feeling it was to know this long trial by fire was nearly over!

Christine had three drains installed during her surgery, and was moving very slowly. Matthew was a little frightened on seeing Mommy so incapacitated, but Jenny was a huge help in assuring him that she was going to be all right. She helped and encouraged all of us.

There was a meeting for Kiwanis I had to attend the evening Christine came home, as I was chairman of the committee that organized an upcoming dinner at the Ronald McDonald House. For those not familiar with the project, the Ronald McDonald House assists families of children with cancer by giving them a place to stay near All Children's Hospital in St. Petersburg. We offered to put on a barbecue and took up a collection for the menu—filet mignon, and hot dogs for children who preferred less sophisticated fare.

I particularly remember a couple with a small child coming up to me with some hesitation as I manned the grill.

"Is it really true that we can each have a filet, and our little girl can have a hot dog?" asked the father.

"Of course," I answered. "She can have a filet, too, if she wants."

Both parents' eyes widened in wonder, then the father asked in a whisper, "What *is* a filet mignon?" They'd never seen one before.

I explained and served them each a steak. About a half hour later, the father came back and asked shyly if he could have another.

I grinned. "Sure! No problem!"

While this event was a break from the stress of caring for Christine, it also provided a graphic glimpse into the lives of other people coping with cancer in the little ones they loved.

Some of the parents told me their stories. One couple told me bluntly that they didn't have much hope, and figured they had come here to watch their child die. It was heartbreaking.

The evening at the Ronald McDonald House was a good one and I was happy to be there, but in another way it was just more of the same agony I knew all too well. If I were to classify my response, I would have to say it warmed my soul. It also reminded me to count my blessings.

That Sunday was Mothers' Day, and Christine was beginning to navigate her way around the house and get her appetite back. She was also complaining about her drains, which gave me some encouragement that she was turning the corner toward recovery. The following Tuesday I took Jenny to the airport and saw her off with a hug, a kiss, and deep thanks for all she had done to see us all through this. On Thursday I took Christine to the doctor, who removed one of the three drains. She began wearing a fanny pack to store the drains so she could move around freely. The pack was almost completely covered by her clothing, which gave me new respect for women's ingenuity. She also wanted to work at least part time that day. What a trooper! Her company, as always, was extremely supportive, and we were all happy to see Christine back in the saddle again.

Within the next three weeks all the drains had been removed, she was back at work almost full-force, and doing well. Despite the discomfort, at least this time we both knew she was cancer-free and headed down the home stretch to recovery.

May 23 was a very happy occasion. Kenny, one of my little brothers in the Big Brothers/Big Sisters program, was graduating from high school and had a basketball scholarship waiting for him, to boot. I drove down to Charlotte High School in Punta Gorda, and was very proud to see him accept his diploma. It was inspiring to see someone who could so easily have become a criminal statistic take the route to success, instead. As I watched the ceremony I remembered the day I had enrolled ten-year-old Kenny and his brother into the Hooked on Phonics Program that had made such a profound difference in their lives, and in mine.

By Saturday, June 8, Christine was much improved, and we decided it was time for a road trip. Since mangoes were now in season, we decided to take a drive down to Pine Island and load up. We continued down the coast to Naples, and went out that night for dinner and shopping. I noticed a tall, wooden heron that had a space in his back for a flowerpot. We went back the next day and brought Harry the Heron home with us, where he joined Jake the Dolphin to become another member of our family.

Chapter 18

A COUPLE OF WEEKS LATER, I suggested we go to a spa for a little pampering. This was a particularly welcome treat for Christine; because of the effects of the radiation treatments, it had been months since she could bear to have her skin touched. Now, she was more than ready for a deep massage and some steam. It turned out to be a great weekend of self-indulgence.

On June 26 we went to lunch at the historic Don CeSar Resort on St. Pete Beach, and booked our wedding there for February 15. We chose the Terrace Room on the fifth floor, which affords a spectacular view of the Gulf of Mexico. That evening we attended a Devil Rays baseball game, and watched it in style in United Banks' private box. To top it all off, the Devil Rays won that night, which was not a frequent occurrence that year. Even though Christine was facing a few more surgeries we were in high spirits. It felt great to have finally set a date for our nuptials.

That Friday we decided it was time to have a party for Erik, Amanda, and Mitchell, all of whom had birthdays coming up. Christine, Matthew, and I took everyone down to the Keys and stayed at a lovely waterfront hotel. We went snorkeling at Pennekamp State Park, booked a fishing charter, and had a ball.

There was another trip I'd been looking forward to: a return to Unity Village. My last visit has been almost a year ago, and I was more than ready for a retreat from the tension. I also signed up for some classes. On July 7, I took a flight to Kansas City and was met again at the airport by a limo driver. As we approached the now-familiar entrance of flowers, the same warm feeling enveloped me: the sense that God was in residence here. I immediately felt at peace and in touch with the positive vibration of this remarkable place.

Check-in and class information were next. Then it was a time to concentrate on meditation, spiritual evolvement, and prayer. I walked over to my favorite place, the Peace Chapel, and spent time giving thanks for what God had done for Christine and me.

The second evening, I took a walk back to the lake where I had first heard the voice. I meditated there until nightfall, feeling more and more certain that everything in my life was falling into place. I rounded a bend on the path on the walk back. There were the deer. The closest ones looked toward me without fear, just as they had before.

"Thank you for bringing me peace a year ago. Thank you for sending me the message that Christine was going to be all right," I whispered into the serene darkness.

I felt the now-familiar conviction that all was going to be

well and continued my trek, then noticed that a foggy mist was forming, just as it had on my previous trip. The same emotions welled up inside me, and the voice I had heard before resonated within me, assuring me once more that Christine was well and that we should go forward with our wedding plans.

My classes began the next day, and I was very impressed with the instructors. They really helped to open my awareness of how lucky I am, how good life really is, and that I should have more of an "attitude of gratitude."

The week went by quickly with more classes, fellowship, prayer, meditation, and progressive spiritual growth. I knew that coming here had played a major role in turning what could have been a great tragedy into an overwhelming triumph for me and my sweetheart.

On Saturday, July 13, I prepared to leave feeling calmer and more blessed by God than I ever had before. This time as the car pulled out of my heaven on earth, I looked back not with a reluctance to leave as I had been last year, but gratitude and happiness in anticipation of what—and who—was waiting for me at home.

The Saturday after my return, Christine and I worked at the annual Care Fair for disadvantaged children. A couple of thousand kids showed up to get their preschool physicals and immunizations, as well as free backpacks. It was very affirming to help so many young lives get off to a healthy start for the school year.

In stark contrast to that pleasant event, later that afternoon Christine and I attended the funeral of one of her friends who had died suddenly a few days ago. As I listened to the service I felt so lucky, so blessed that my Christine was still with me and on the way to full recovery. I reflected how it could very well have been she we were eulogizing, instead of celebrating her continued existence in this world. Tears of gratitude to God filled my eyes as I glanced at her.

The following week, there was a notice at our local City Hall that they were looking for people to give blood. With my renewed revelation at Unity Village and the sad contrast of the recent funeral fresh in my mind, donating the gift of life seemed like one of the best things I could do. I went to the big Bloodmobile in the parking lot and had my blood pressure checked; the reading was normal, though lately it had been a bit high. It felt good to give a little something back to the medical profession that had helped my sweetheart make it through the valley of the shadow.

As the calendar approached August 2, we prepared ourselves for Christine's surgery—the sixth in eighteen months. They were going to reconstruct her other breast and do more work on the irradiated side that had been so damaged. Unfortunately, there was no Jenny to help us this time.

Christine had to be at the hospital at 6:30 AM (why can't they schedule these things at a reasonable hour?). I took Matthew out for breakfast and then to school before heading for the hospital to wait for what the surgeon had told me would be at least an 8-hour procedure. Since I knew from prior experience that I would be useless at work, I did some errands around town before picking up Matthew that afternoon. I forced myself not to dwell on what could go wrong and tried to keep a positive attitude, but it was difficult.

I never could stand hospitals, even before I met Christine. Heck, I don't even watch medical shows on television. I've learned that when I'm in that anxious state of waiting that I should keep to myself, since my patience runs a bit thin. In other words, it's best for me and everyone else if I stay busy and keep my mouth shut.

During the countless hours I've spent in hospital waiting rooms, I've noticed that most people spend their time watching daytime television. Personally, I can't stand watching these inane dramas and listening to people argue about who has been unfaithful to whom—especially when the woman I'm devoted to is on the operating table. I think it would be much better to take out the TVs and play some soft music, with videos available to give people a hopeful look at how to be a better caregiver: not a dismal view of the seamier side of life.

But the time finally passed, and it was time to pick up Matthew from preschool. I dropped him off at his dad's house and went back to wait some more at the hospital. The doctor came out around 5:00 PM and let me know that Christine had come through everything like the champion she was, and was recovering well in post-op. He said she would still be unconscious for a while, but that as soon as she started coming around the nurses would let me into the recovery room to see her.

I certainly wasn't going to hang around that horror of a waiting room, so I left to get a bite to eat. They let me in to see Christine when I returned a couple of hours later. She was hooked up to a lot of monitors, and still very groggy, I alternated between the bedside where I tried to be comforting during her brief conscious moments, then walking to the nurse's station for updates on her condition. I know I must have driven every nurse on the floor nuts; if any of the machines attached to Christine made even the slightest sound, I pressed the call button or hurried down the hall and demanded immediate attention.

Each of them told me the same thing. "Don't worry, Mr. Allard…it's okay. Everything is going just fine. There's absolutely nothing to worry about."

It took quite some time before I believed them. After they

had to deal with me, I realized anew why nurses deserve the title "angels of mercy."

After a few hours of this, the staff rather strongly insisted that I go home and get some rest. Utterly punchy with exhaustion by now, I didn't need much convincing.

I went back to my house and my good friend Dimitri came over with another buddy, Jerry. It was a good thing Jerry drove a cab for a living, because Dimitri and I decided we needed to go out and blow off a little steam; a designated driver was an absolute necessity. Dimitri and Jerry were very patient with me, and let me vent all I needed about Christine's surgeries and the frustration of constant waiting. I started to wind down after a couple of drinks and became more philosophical. I also remembered that its times like these when your friends are such a blessing.

Chapter 19

THE NEXT DAY, AUGUST 3, I got up and telephoned the hospital to check on Christine's condition. They told me she was a little more coherent, and that they were waiting for the doctor to come in to see her on morning rounds. It was a great relief to hear my sweetheart's voice.

I would have liked to have given her a greeting in person, but I was going to have to go paddle my own canoe...literally. I was heading an outing for the Kiwanis group that day and a canoe trip was about the last thing I wanted to do, but Christine was adamant.

"Bill, there's nothing you can do for me here right now," she said emphatically. "I know you love me and want to be here, and that's what really matters. Go ahead and take the trip. You can't let all those people down, and it might do you some good to get out for a while." She laughed. "Don't worry...I'll still be here when you get back—and maybe by then I can even get out of this place!"

So Dimitri and I went off to meet the group at the Hillsborough River. After canoeing for a while and looking at the beauty of nature with my friends, I began to relax a bit. I knew Christine had been right to urge me to go. The more I got in touch with my feelings while I was gliding over the water, the more certain I felt that she was truly going to be all right.

I began to review the logistics. Matthew would be coming back from his father's house on Monday when school would begin, Christine would need a lot of help once she came home, and I still had a company to run.

Well, I told myself, *you'd better face the fact that there's a lot of work ahead after she gets home. And this time, Jenny won't be here to help.*

I paddled on, newly appreciative of the fact that this might be my last chance to enjoy a stress-free environment for a while—and that environment was really something to see. We must have sighted twenty alligators that day, hundreds of birds, turtles...all glorying in the beautiful ecosystem that is Florida. By the time we got everyone off the river and enjoying their lunch, it was mid-afternoon. I said my farewells as quickly as I could without seeming rude and rushed to the hospital.

Christine was still being put through some procedures that were preventing her from coming home. We watched TV and did some reading until about 7:00 PM, when they finally released her.

It was a little difficult getting Christine into the house, since I didn't have Jenny to help with lifting and getting her settled in bed. There was a restaurant within walking distance of our house called Patrick's, so I ordered some soup she liked and dinner for myself, then hurried over to pick it up. This began a new phase of caregiving I hadn't explored before. Christine had been independent and relatively functional during her earlier procedures; after this surgery, she couldn't even go to the bathroom alone, much less dress or bathe herself.

She had a pretty good weekend resting at home, and slept a lot. This gave me time to take to run errands, clean house, and make what business calls I could.

That Monday, Matthew came home from his dad's house, I took him to school, and then went back home to take care of Christine. Once I had her settled for an afternoon nap, I took a run downtown to the office for a couple of hours, picked Matthew up from school, and we headed home so I could start dinner. While the three of us living together as a family was a happy time, there was still a lot of tension in the atmosphere. Matthew was stressed because Mommy had drains coming out of her again—even more of them. She wasn't feeling up to doing her usual motherly things, which concerned him. It was heartrending to see the anxiety in that little boy's face.

But by Wednesday, Christine was already beginning to feel stronger. By the following Monday, August 12, she was back working part-time. She did this, by the way, with four drains leading down to the fanny pack discreetly hidden under her clothes. Ten days ago, she had been on an operating table, and now she was back at work. What an amazing woman!

Another two weeks went by. On Friday, August 23, the last of the detested drains were removed, largely due to Christine's insistence. She had to go on a business trip to Philadelphia on the 26th, and those tubes were *not* coming along. Though she still couldn't lift anything heavy, my assistance was becoming less and less necessary. She was elated to be drain-free, and

I saw her off at the airport with a smile; she was obviously happy to be back at the work she loved.

About a month after Christine's surgery, we attended a wedding at St. Simon's Island on the coast of Georgia. Although it was a six-hour drive from St. Petersburg, it was definitely worth it. We stopped in Gainesville on the way (home of the Florida Gators). Erik had lived there for a while and I knew the beautiful campus town pretty well, so I decided to take my beloved to a local restaurant that featured rack of lamb. We ventured on to Georgia and checked into the resort to get some sleep, since the wedding was the next morning.

This event promised to be more interesting than most. Christine had a friend whose son was getting married. What made it interesting was that her friend was gay and not everyone knew it. He had been married at one time to the son's mother, but lived with his lover now.

Christine asked him, "What does your son and the rest of your family think about your being gay, and openly having your lover here?"

He smiled gently at Christine and answered softly, "They don't know."

We both looked at him in amazement, then the three of us laughed.

Actually, the only other one who knew was the ex-wife, who wasn't about to mention it to anyone. In fact, it seemed to me during the reception that she might even be making a play for her former husband.

As I said, the drive was definitely worth it.

The following day we enjoyed some R& R at Jekyll Island, swam in the Atlantic, and then took a ferry over to Jacksonville, just over the Florida/Georgia border. We brought along a cooler and filled it with all kinds of seafood from the dockside markets. It was the first time since the last surgery that we were both healthy and in the mood to have fun.

September 4, 2002: time to celebrate my birthday. Our first stop was for dinner at a new local restaurant in town called Perch, which had received good reviews in the paper. From there we went to a Devil Rays baseball game. Christine was in great spirits, feeling good, and it was a great occasion.

A couple of days later, Christine, Matthew, Mitchell, and I all got involved in National Beach Cleanup Day on our own St. Pete Beach. As the title implies, the tradition involves citizens cleaning up the mess left on our beautiful beaches by thoughtless litterbugs.

Even though she was still recovering, Christine was out there with the rest of the volunteers picking up trash and setting her son Matthew a great example of civic responsibility, as well as personal courage. The following day we all had a great outing at Busch Gardens in Tampa on the roller coasters and spent the day in family love, harmony, and laughter.

Another week or so later, on October 5, Matthew had his sixth birthday party at Chuckie Cheese. The party consisted of nine of his friends, so we had ten children to handle between the ages of three and eight years old. The cuisine consists of pizza and other child-oriented snack foods that would make the late Dr. Atkins turn over in his non-carbohydrate grave, but the kids loved it. So did we. The real attraction, however, was the floor show. At timed intervals, the larger-than-life cartoon characters of Mr. Cheese's world came miraculously and loudly to life in a loud musical interlude that seemed to last forever.

Some good friends of ours from England arrived about a week later. We took them along with some other friends on a cruise up the Intracoastal Waterway. The trip took about an hour, and then it was off to the Salt Rock Grill for an incredible lunch. Another surgery for Christine was looming on the horizon, and that afternoon did a lot toward taking her mind off health concerns and putting it on just enjoying the moment.

The following weekend we took another trip to Gainesville to watch the University of Florida Gators play Auburn University. I got into an impromptu basketball match with some of the students on campus before kickoff. Christine was an excellent cheerleader and my team actually beat the students, which was hard for even me to believe.

I could hear them grumbling as they walked away, "Boy, I can't believe that old man beat us."

Needless to say, this "old man" was very pleased, and Christine was quite proud of her star athlete. We made our way to The Swamp, and watched a great game in which the Gators beat Auburn. I grinned all the way home, relishing the fact that Christine was with me and feeling well, and that I still had it in me to show kids half my age a thing or two about basketball.

Chapter 20

IT WAS FRIDAY, OCTOBER 25, 2002: the date for Christine's seventh surgery in twenty-two months. But by that time, who was counting?

Words can't describe how relieved I was that this was the last operation. I knew the whole experience had taken quite a toll on me; my nerves, my patience, my entire being was being beat up by too much time in the world of medicine and sickness. My mental stability was starting to crumble a bit.

Matthew and I took Christine to the hospital very early in the morning. We dropped her off at Outpatient Surgery, because this procedure wasn't going to require an overnight stay. This was going to be only about a three-hour surgery, and she was scheduled to be ready to go home by five that afternoon.

I took Matthew out for breakfast, where we talked about Mommy's operation over eggs and toast. Convinced that he was handling the situation well, I dropped him off at his school and made it back to the hospital about 8:00 AM, just in time to meet the surgeon. He told me Christine was prepped and that they were getting ready to wheel her into the OR. He advised me to relax and check back in about eleven. I was allowed in to give Christine a kiss, told her I knew she'd be fine, and tried to ignore the gut-wrenching fear as she was taken through the double doors to go under yet another scalpel. I felt a physical pain in my heart as I saw her going yet another ordeal. No matter how many times the physicians assured me everything was going to be all right, there was always some concern in the back of my mind.

What if something goes wrong? I thought, *what if the voice I heard was just my wishful imagination?*

I felt a tremor vibrate through my whole body as I sat down to await the outcome, then decided to review the latest test findings from the oncologist in an attempt to calm my doubts. Her tumor markers were low, there was no sign that the cancer was back, and today was the end of Christine's reconstruction. This should be a happy surgery, if there is such a thing—but I was as scared I was the first time I sat in a hospital waiting room. It was just another sign to me that I was worn out and my emotional control was at an all-time low.

I left to run some errands, as I usually did while awaiting the outcome. My mind was so scattered that even today I can't remember where I went or what I did. I was just trying to avoid the inevitable trashy daytime programs in the waiting room.

When I returned to the hospital at eleven, I was told there would be at least a half-hour wait. There was. The surgeon finally came out.

"She's okay," he said simply. His smile said it all. "Everything went just fine, and she looks just as great as we all hoped.

She should be ready to go home in a few hours. Why don't you leave and go about your business, then come back around three? She's in Recovery right now, and there's really nothing you can do here."

I thanked him profusely, rode the elevator down to the lobby, walked out to my car, sat down in the driver's seat, and began to cry with happiness, joy, and incredible belief that it was over. Christine was better. She had survived cancer.

I had to sit there for about ten minutes before I could compose myself. As soon as I could drive, I went somewhere for lunch—I don't remember where, then killed more time by having the oil changed in my car.

By then, it was time to pick up Matthew. As I drove him to his father's house, I explained that Mommy was doing just fine. Then, it was finally time to go back to the hospital. But I didn't have to wait to get there to hear her voice. She called me on my cell phone.

"Where are you?" she demanded. "I am *so* ready to get out of here!"

I laughed as I made my way back to Christine; that was my sweetheart, all right.

When I got to her room, she was already trying to pack her things. The nurse got a wheelchair (mandatory for all patients, even if all you have is an ingrown toenail), and off we went to the car. She was very sore in various places, but you'd never have known it from the smile on her face.

To say that Christine was happy to be home was an understatement. I got out the menu from the always dependable Patrick's (kind of our local version of the TV series *Cheers*), called in our dinner order, and walked over to pick it up. While waiting for our food, I had a cocktail and talked to some of the locals who were well aware of Christine's condition and were eager for the latest update.

"It's a good thing we're at the end of this trail," I laughed a little ruefully, "because I'm also about at the end of my rope."

Our friends smiled in understanding, and happiness that what could have been such a tragedy was nearing a happy conclusion. It was a real relief for me to have such a sympathetic audience, and I was able to let go of some of the tension by talking about all the events of the past twenty-two months. After all, a lot had happened from slipping a diamond on Christine's finger to holding her hand through two long rounds of eight chemotherapy treatments, thirty-five radiation treatments, and seven surgeries.

Everyone could see my nerves were frayed, and I was still a bit in shock. They bought me another drink. I sipped it until the food was ready, then thanked everyone and took dinner home to my sweetheart. After our meal, she said that she was still quite sore and was ready to go to bed. I tucked her in and we both called it a night. As I lay there in bed, I thanked God from my heart that she was okay, and that we were home at last.

Christine rested on Friday, all Saturday and Sunday, and needed a little help getting around. I took Monday and Tuesday off to care for her, and by the following Wednesday she was back at work.

It was time to pick up Matthew from Tom's house (Matthew's dad), where he had been staying during those first painful days of Christine's recovery. I had to take the little guy to school, since Tom had no car, professed he didn't have a job, and didn't pay child support. It fell to me to chauffeur Matthew to these paternal visits; I kept my feelings about the man to myself. After all, Tom was Matthew's father, and this affectionate, giving little boy loved him. Daddy may have been just a step above useless, but it didn't matter to his child, even on those days when he was supposed to see a father who was "unavailable." Tom never seemed to want his son around much, especially if the child was sick, so the majority of parental influence fell to Christine and me.

After I dropped Matthew off at school, I went about my business and cared for Christine until it was time to pick her son up. Yes, it had been a long ordeal, and her ex-husband had not been much help. Despite the frustration, I had become quite adept at keeping a smile on my face and my comments to a minimum.

Christine had a doctor's appointment on Tuesday. She got a good report and was told that she was healing well, but needed to rest. After we saw the doctor I went to pick up Matthew from school, and the three of us had dinner at home. Then I took Matthew back to school for the Pumpkin Carving Party that night to celebrate Halloween. We picked up a nice, big pumpkin at the grocery store on the way there, and had a great time with this time-honored activity of carving a big squash into a scary face. His teacher was really getting into it, digging in with both hands into the pumpkins to bring out all the pulp and seeds (the kids found that part wonderfully "yucky"). She asked Matthew if he'd like to take the pumpkin guts home and spread it on his toast in the morning, which he found very funny.

On the drive home from school, we had a little talk about how Mommy was doing. I assured him that she was getting much better, but wasn't up to being jumped on and rough-housing quite yet.

"She just needs a little rest, Matthew," I explained. "But in a little while, she's going to be okay."

He smiled at that, and it was a joyful, hopeful evening for both of us.

Christine went back to work on October 30, which would have seemed surprising from anyone but my own bionic woman. She started off with just a couple of hours a day, but was bringing herself up to speed as quickly as she could. The first evening after her return to the office she was feeling strong enough to keep Matthew by herself, so I went to a meeting at our church. I had become a facilitator for a discussion group at our church. I found the fellowship stimulating, and it was a good and inspiring break from the stress of constant health and child care. I even vented a bit to the group about how tired I was of the unrelenting pressure and twenty-two months of worry that had basically knocked the stuffing out of me.

The group was very friendly and supportive, and shared some of their own experiences in an attempt to let me know how well they understood. I was told it was okay to be tired; it was all right to be worn out, and it was certainly understandable that I was still in shock from it all.

Christine went back to the office the next day for a few more hours, and within a few days was back to a full-time schedule. On Saturday, November 9, the two of us began working diligently on our wedding plans, since February 15th was only three months away. We took a trip to Dillard's department store and had a wonderful time at the bridal registry, then discussed more details about the kind of ceremony and reception we wanted.

The next week Christine went off to a day-into-evening business meeting, and Matthew and I were on our own. We visited a book fair at school, where pizza was served to give a little incentive to education. We bought a book, a CD, a learning game, and Matthew had his first taste of chocolate pizza. This was a big hit, and we had a lot of fun.

Bear in mind, we had reached this point of resuming a normal life only eighteen days since Christine's last surgery. Whoever called women "the weaker sex" had obviously never met my fiancée.

On November 17, we formally joined the Unity Christ Church we'd been attending for some time, and it was a joyous experience for us both. That evening we celebrated by attending a Sierra Club fundraiser. We had a nice dinner at the Florida Aquarium and an auction where we bid on various items, but we spent most of the time talking about our wedding. I thanked God in my heart as I walked beside this remarkable woman, and was amazed anew at what His grace can do to change lives.

The following Tuesday, Christine was very busy at work and getting home later than usual, so I agreed to take Matthew to the PTA meeting at his school. The school's curriculum was fundamental, with excellent programs that required a lot of parental participation. This meant attending PTA was mandatory, not voluntary, I found it very informative, and had a good time meeting the other parents and seeing how Matthew was doing in school.

On Thursday, November 21, Erik and Amanda went to Chicago for Erik's ten-year high school reunion. Mitchell and Haley were left in our care while Christine and I stayed at their house, and I made sure to adjust my schedule to include a lot of family outings. We went to the beach museum, Ronald McDonald Land, a boat show, Chuckie Cheese (of course), and a Christmas tree show. Matthew joined us when his schedule permitted, and it was wonderful to see the way our extended family was coming together.

On Saturday we were relieved of babysitting duty by Amanda's parents, Barbara and Paul. They arrived in St. Pete and took the kids for Saturday and Sunday. On Sunday night, Christine and I took over again and brought the children to the Great Explorations Museum the next day. Haley was about one year old and not quite potty trained yet, and a child came out of the big snake model at the museum with a quizzical look on his face.

"Something smells stinky in there," he announced to the general public.

I saw Haley follow him out, picked her up, and noticed her training pants were soaked. Further research revealed that there was a lot more than "number one" involved. Talk about Grandpa duties! There's no delicate way to put it; poop was everywhere. It took quite a while to get our little princess freshened up, but that's where my experience as a dad really came in handy.

Erik and Amanda returned that evening with glowing reports about how much fun the reunion was, and we brought them up to date on how great the kids had been.

Reverend Ron and his wife, Amy, came to the house for dinner and to discuss our wedding vows. It was now less than 90 days before the big day. To those of you who have planned such an event, you know how little time that is to get everything together. We barbecued salmon for our guests and enjoyed a great meal while talking about this very significant event in our lives. Things went very smoothly, and we all had a nice time. Christine was feeling particularly well that evening, and

I was really starting to get into the joy of planning our upcoming wedding.

The next Thursday was Thanksgiving, and we celebrated with a nice turkey at home with our happy family. We had a lot to be thankful for: that Christine had come through her cancer encounter, that we had kept our faith and believed that God was going to heal her, and that He had somehow helped me in helping her. The surgeries were over, the wounds were healed, and the time for our nuptials had finally arrived.

While we were in the midst of our own plans, we attended the marriage of two dear friends of ours, Dale and Sarah. Since Reverend Ron was going to be officiating, Christine and I thought this was a great chance to see our minister in action. We were both very pleased at what we witnessed. As we danced at the happy couple's reception, we smiled at the thought that our own wedding was only two months away.

The following Friday, December 6, we went to the Stouffer Vinoy Resort to hear a band play that we were thinking about for our reception. They were playing a party there and we loved their music, so we struck up a conversation with them during a break. They seemed really enthused about playing for us at the Don Cesar, so it looked like the music was at least one item we could strike off our list of things to do.

December 11 was the day Christine had set for her office Christmas party, which would be held in our home in Punta Vista this year. She was very busy getting everything together, which was quite a job (the guest list ran up to 45 people). She did an outstanding job, and it was one of the happiest Christmas parties I've ever attended. We played the piano, sang Christmas carols and other favorite songs, and had a grand, old-fashioned celebration of thankfulness.

The next Friday night was my office Christmas party, which

was held again at the Vinoy. In spite of all our trials and tribulations my business had done well, which is why we were able to afford such a lavish party. From the moment we arrived for an exquisite gourmet dinner, the resort did a standup job. The band they had that night was great, Christine looked fabulous, and we talked about how blessed we were and what a change it was from last year, when all we had to hold on to was hope.

Christine and I went to a Murder Mystery Dinner Theater the following evening, which was great fun. The next day, the church had their Christmas party. After that we went off to a movie and dinner to have some time alone together. It had been quite an eventful holiday calendar!

The next thing I knew, it was December 23. Could it possibly be Christmas already? To make this particular holiday even more exciting, it was only seven weeks until our wedding.

On Christmas Eve, the whole family was due to assemble for one of my now-famous salmon grills. Erik and Amanda were coming with Mitchell and Haley, Our good friend Dimitri was attending, of course, and we had a multitude of other friends and family that made for a memorable evening. We also exchanged gifts, which added to a truly merry Christmas Eve.

On Christmas Day, we spent much of the day relaxing at home. We went to Erik and Amanda's house that evening to see them and the grandkids. Amanda's parents and grandparents were also there for a family gathering that was an equally joyous celebration.

Chapter 21

A WEEK LATER, IT WAS New Year's Eve. Christine and I decided that even with all the excitement of the upcoming wedding, we would give Erik and Amanda time off for a date and take Mitchell and Haley for a sleepover at our house. We cooked up dinner for all three kids (Matthew was thrilled, of course), and let those who could stay up for the big countdown to midnight. It was not a sad thing for Christine and I to see 2002 expire; we were looking forward to a better 2003.

The evening was kind of a tradeoff for us. At 10:00 AM on New Year's morning, we dropped the kids off (including Matthew) back with Erik and Amanda. Christine and I got back in the car and headed for the Outback Bowl, a yearly college football game in Tampa. The Gators were in the bowl that year and Christine was very excited, but they lost to Michigan. We still had a great time. Afterward, we went to the home of Christine's friends, Jeanne and Jim, who were also throwing a New Year's Day football bash.

January 2 was "pro-environment" day at our house with the purchase of a hybrid electric car. This new Honda hybrid meant trading in my Honda Accord, The sting of parting with a car I already liked was lessened by the fact that this new baby could get up to 50 miles per gallon.

Our appointment at Sacino's Formal Wear was later that week. Christine came along to manage Matthew and give me positive feedback, while Matthew and Erik were there to be fitted for their own tuxedoes. One thing the trio of wedding males agreed on was that we wanted our tuxedoes to match. We chose a vested, Pierce-Brosnan-as-James-Bond kind of look that made us all happy.

The pre-wedding festivities were beginning to pile up quickly. On January 8, Christine and I spent a lot of time going over the guest list. Though the invitations had been mailed some time ago, we hadn't gone over the R.S.V.P.s yet.

Though we were having great fun I remember asking her at one point, "So, how are you feeling?" I guess the idea of someone you love living with cancer isn't a mindset that disappears overnight.

I could tell from Christine's smile that she understood. She looked into my eyes and replied emphatically, "Bill, I feel terrific! I'm so excited about our wedding and the clean bill of health from my doctors, aren't you?" She laughed with sheer joy; I loved the sound of it. "I'm well again, do you hear me? *I'm well!*"

I grinned, acknowledged her inarguable point, and told myself to stop being so paranoid. After that, we just passed the afternoon in happy anticipation of the happy upcoming union.

On January 13, Christine and I took a little stroll down to the County Building; it seemed a nice day to get a marriage license. From there we went to our ring fittings. Pat Kelly is a great guy who works at Silverberg's, a family of jewelers revered as one of the town's respected, genteel dynasties for decades. He knew our whole story by now, and was very excited and happy for us.

After the final fittings and a lot of handshakes all around, Christine and I went to lunch. We smiled at each other blissfully over the table, happy that all the papers were in order, all the fittings had been done, and that soon we would be walking down the aisle.

A couple of days later we had one of our workers come over to pressure clean the house, do some touch-up painting, and my wife-to-be had a whole list of other "honey-dos." We wanted our home to look its best when we began our new life as a married couple.

A week later, on January 22, we decided to use a Christmas present from Erik and Amanda: a Starship Cruise out of Tampa. This wasn't one of your hot-dog-and-soda cruises, either. We had a nice dinner with plenty of *vino*, and the atmosphere was quite romantic. Our happiness and desire burned like a flame as we held each other and watched the moonlight dance across Tampa Bay.

It was now less than a month before the wedding, and I'll be the first to admit I was becoming a little nervous. During this time I got some help by seeing Eva, our massage therapist, who helped me relax. I also saw Shirley, the nurse who handled my elevated blood pressure. Then there was George, our chiropractor, who did his best to keep me balanced and stress-free.

On January 30, we had to phone the Don CeSar with the final number of guests who would be at the reception. As I recall, when Christine and I initially planned this event we thought about a hundred would be adequate; when we got to the final tally, that was exactly what we had. What a beautiful reception it was going to be!

February arrived and it was high time for a break from all the nuptial planning, so we took another ride together up to Gainesville. This time the game was Gator basketball, and the opponent was Arkansas. We had great seats and a wonderful dinner after the game.

By February 9, things were getting really close to the wire. We spent some time working on table seating, which is an art form in itself. Our first out of town guests were already arriving: Tim and Evelyn from London. They had just arrived from Wimbledon, and were full of delightful tales of England at its best. Their arrival was only the beginning of an influx of people that made me realize just how complicated planning a wedding can be.

Christine and I had also been looking at homes lately, since our new, extended family seemed a bit cramped for my two-bedroom house. On Tuesday, February 11, just four days before the ceremony, we finalized the deal on a four-bedroom, two-bath home in Tierra Verde (a lovely area not far from the Don Cesar). There was a big family room, a huge master bedroom, swimming pool, and hot tub. It just seemed like the perfect wedding gift for my lovely bride: a place we could begin our marriage in a completely new environment free of all associations with illness.

In short, I wanted a new, healthy home for my new, healthy Christine.

That was accomplished by Tuesday, February 11. On

Wednesday, my brother Joe and his wife, Alicia, arrived. We spent the day taking them out on the boat, and my mother arrived that evening to join us. Christine's sister and her family came next, Dimitri, Erik, the children…well, there was nothing I could do but grill salmon for everyone.

On Thursday, February 13, we had a pre-wedding golf outing. About eleven showed up, and we had a lot of fun. After golf, we drove to Sacino's to meet Matthew and Christine and pick up our tuxedoes.

We proceeded to Patrick's Restaurant, where a dozen people were meeting us for dinner. My daughter Kellie and her new beau, Kraig, were there, and this was my first opportunity to meet him. In fact, this had been the first chance we'd had to introduce these wonderful people in our lives to one another, and it was a joy to watch the interaction.

The next day was a Valentine's Day canoe trip. A group of us met at Hillsborough River State Park, a lovely place just filled with wildlife and birds. We saw about twenty alligators, too, which keeps one reminded to have a healthy respect for nature.

What is even more exciting than seeing an alligator, however, is navigating around one in a canoe. Let's just say that it adds quite a bit to the excitement. Christine and I were in one canoe, and there was about fifteen of us canoeing that day. It was a three-hour trip, and the thrills of the alligators, the ever-changing light on the water, and the color of the Roseate Spoonbills made the world seem like Eden.

We had the wedding rehearsal dinner that evening, hosted by my son Erik at his home. About twenty people were there, and a caterer from an Italian restaurant wined and dined us exquisitely.

Talking about the wedding the next day amid the love of

family and friends was a feeling I know neither Christine nor I will ever forget. That party was a ten on a one-to-ten scale of happiness.

Chapter 22

IT WAS SATURDAY, FEBRUARY 15: our wedding day. It was hard to believe that it was barely two years ago that we had become engaged. I woke up that morning with a tremendous feeling of excitement.

Christine and I each had numerous things to take care of, so I whisked Matthew away to meet my daughter Kellie, her boyfriend Kraig, and numerous other family members at the Seaside Grill, a neat little breakfast spot right on the seashore. We had a great meal while discussing the upcoming day. Kellie already knew about my present to Christine—a new house— and wanted to see it. We took a quick ride over there and pulled up in front to see the current owner working in his garden. He graciously allowed us inside, and Matthew was particularly excited to see his new home. Kellie loved it, too. Shortly afterward, she and Kraig left.

The next part of the day's plan was a 1:00 PM meeting with Erik at the ceremony site: the beach in front of Hurley Park, where there was a lovely gazebo. On a more practical note, there were also bathrooms and a shelter in case the weather took a turn for the worse. The ceremony was planned to begin at 5:00 PM, which meant that the sun would be close to setting just as we took our vows. We walked across the small wooden crosswalk toward the dunes, and picked out a location that seemed to command the best view. In fact, our backdrop toward the shore side was a church. We were still close enough to the water so that the sound of the waves would be heard clearly on our wedding video. We even policed the area by picking up stray beer cans and throwing them in the trash.

By the time we finished, it was around 2:00 PM. Since Erik was my best man, he planned to arrive in his tuxedo at about 4:00 to let the photographers and guests know where everything would be set up. We said our farewells and parted ways. The limousine was fetching him around 3:30, and then picking up the mother of the bride and groom so that family would be on hand to greet the arriving guests.

I went home with Matthew and got him started with his pre-wedding grooming, then began getting dressed myself.

Then, Christine walked in the door.

She looked amazing. Her hair looked just beautiful, and every moment she spent at the salon had been more than worth it. There were flowers interwoven with her hairstyle; she laughed and said they called it "wedding hair."

Her arrival relieved me of the responsibility of Matthew for a little while, so I took advantage of the opportunity to run up to Sandros, the gentleman who cuts my hair. I made it in about 3:30, and he did a superlative job of blow-drying and styling my hair so the wind wouldn't mess it up too much as we stood on the beach.

I was back at the house by 4:00 and donned my tux while Christine was putting on her wedding gown. The phone rang; it was Jerry, our limo driver who had also been our designated driver on my recent outing with Dimitri. Jerry assured us that things were on schedule.

The next thing I knew, the limo was in front of the house. Though I wasn't completely dressed yet, I walked outside to greet Jerry as he headed toward our door.

He looked me up and down. "Hey, what's up?" he demanded jovially, "everyone's already there waiting for you—including the reverend—and you aren't even dressed yet!"

I looked at my watch: it was 4:45. Where had the time gone?

I spotted our next door neighbors, Scott and Karen, eyeing us curiously from their yard. They'd been invited to the wedding but were waiting for their cab to arrive; it was clear that they'd been doing a little pre-celebrating.

I grinned. "Well, we've got this big limo here to take us to the ceremony, so you might as well ride along with us." I said. "I'm sure you can catch a ride to the reception with someone once we all get there."

"Sure!" they announced. "Wait a second...we'll go get a bottle of champagne!"

There we were, drinking champagne out in the front yard with our limo driver. It occurred to me that perhaps I should get back in the house and finish dressing for my wedding. The trio stayed behind and made more toasts to our happiness.

I opened the door to see Matthew, who was all dressed up in his tuxedo. Then, my eyes went to Christine. Words can't describe how beautiful she was.

"I'm ready," she said simply.

As for me, I was still speechless at her loveliness. I immediately got the rest of my tux on and opened the door for her and Matthew, and we made our way out to the limo. It was now 5:10. Jerry and our neighbor, Scott, looked at Christine and said in unison, "Oh, my God!"

It was an apt tribute. We drank a little more champagne in the front yard, then finally got into the limo to find a little surprise left for us by my son: a bottle of Dom Perignon in an ice bucket, along with some crystal flutes. This was hailed with great glee, and we rode away in high spirits.

Fortunately, we were only ten minutes away from the ceremony site. Scott and Karen jumped out first, and then I stepped out with Matthew.

Erik was already at my side. "Hey, Dad, everyone's ready to go!"

I followed his pointing finger down the beach and saw what looked like a small army waiting for us in a huge circle: a formation we thought would make the ceremony a little more intimate.

Walking over the small wooden crosswalk toward the dunes wasn't nearly as easy or graceful in dress shoes, but I forgot the discomfort when I saw that the sand had been decorated with thousands of flower petals all the way from the limousine, over the crosswalk, all the way to the place we had chosen for the ceremony.

The videographer and photographers were snapping pictures everywhere, and it felt like the red carpet at the Academy Awards.

"Look over here!" one photographer shouted.

"Let's have another smile like that!" exclaimed another.

"Who's the other couple?" someone asked.

I laughed and told them that they were guests who just rode along with us, and weren't part of the wedding party.

Erik sent everyone down to the seaside with the authority of George S. Patton, then turned to me and asked calmly, "Ready to go, Dad?"

Erik, my best man, and Jenny, Christine's sister and maid of honor, linked arms and headed toward the crowd. I followed, and took in all the smiling faces of our friends and family as I headed for my position at Erik's side in front of Reverend Ron. Though we had made it clear on our wedding invitations that the occasion was "black tie optional," it amazed and touched me that so many of our friends had chosen to honor us by showing up in their very best.

I saw everyone look past me, and turned to see Matthew escorting his mother down the sandy, petal-strewn aisle. The image of that little boy bringing his beautiful mother to marry me is one I shall never forget. The crowd gasped at how stunning and happy she looked, and I beamed with pride and happiness.

Christine took her place next to me in front of the minister, and Reverend Ron began the ceremony. My wife-to-be had written our vows (with a little input from me, but not much), and they were as inspiring as they were poetic. As we made our solemn promises to each other and reached the part where we said, "I do," flocks of doves and seagulls appeared suddenly and began to fly around us. When I saw them in the photos later, it reminded me of the experience I had witnessed among the deer at Unity Village. It was if God had sent these birds to our ceremony to emphasize His blessing upon us, and to remind me of the miracle of Christine's healing.

I am here, too, He seemed to say.

We exchanged our rings as the birds hovered about us, and

when Reverend Ron said, "You may kiss the bride," I didn't need to be told twice.

Applause broke out as our minister presented "Mr. and Mrs. William Allard," and we were immediately engulfed by swarms of loving people.

After another round of photographs, it was time to head for the reception at the Don CeSar. Christine, Matthew and I got back in the limousine for a short, two-mile trip to the resort. Jerry beeped the horn all during our drive while Christine and I finished off what was left of the Dom Perignon. Matthew beamed from ear-to-ear.

The videographer and photographers were waiting for us at the Don, and filmed us as we made our way to the fifth floor and the Terrace Room. Our guests were there as well, enjoying champagne and appetizers. We even managed to get a few more photos on the veranda before the sun finally set. The Don did their usual five-star catering, the band we'd hired was great, and we enjoyed dancing and holding each other close among those we love the most.

One of our friends, Russell, had brought his son, Joe. He and Matthew were just a couple of years apart, and they had a wonderful time playing at the celebration.

One of the photographers reported to me that she had asked Matthew what he thought of the wedding. She got a great shot of his answer: a thumbs-up and a huge grin. It is one of our favorite photos of our happy day.

Jenny came over the following morning to pick up Matthew; Christine and I were off for our honeymoon cruise to Ecuador and the Galapagos Islands. We snorkeled with the abundant sea life and enjoyed the unspoiled beauty of the islands while staying on the *Santa Cruz*, a 90-passenger yacht with service that even Ari Onassis would have approved. Since we were the only honeymoon couple on this trip, they gave us particular attention.

When we finally returned from paradise, it was to prepare for the move to our new home. Christine was not planning to work full-time much longer at her office; she wanted to begin devoting more time to helping other families cope with cancer, putting to work what we had both learned during her ordeal.

One area she noticed that needs special attention are the children of cancer victims. While everyone is involved in caring for the patient, who is taking care of the kids? Who's taking them to soccer practice, or helping them with their homework? Who is making sure they had as normal a life as possible while Mommy or Daddy is going through medical treatments?

As Christine told me, "If I hadn't had the support group of you and all my friends and family, what would I have done? What about all those nightmare stories we heard in the hospitals and treatment facilities about people who had no one at all to help them?"

The doctors told us a sad fact; when a woman gets breast cancer, more often than not the husband leaves because he can't deal with the difficulties and disfigurement involved.

Christine had even come up with a name for her concept: Angels for Children of Fighters. While we don't know yet just how widely this plan will be implemented, my wife has already found a way to introduce it with a local oncology group. This, she says, is her way of paying back all those who helped her, and of helping those who will someday have to climb the same mountain she did. This was remarkable to hear from a woman who was told there was a sixty percent chance she would be dead within two years of her initial diagnosis. She beat the odds, and wanted to help other people beat them, too.

As I end this story, we are living happily ever after in our new home. I have hesitated to tell anyone about my experiences at Unity Village. However, I also feel the need to share this story with others dealing with doubts about their ability to cope with the stress of cancer in someone they love.

Thank you, God. Thank you, Silent Unity and Unity Village; you were the catalyst that healed my love, and put our lives back together.

Amen.

www.ingramcontent.com/pod-product-compliance
Lightning Source LLC
Chambersburg PA
CBHW051425280526
45785CB00003B/1164